Longevity Training-Book 3 –Enable Your Life Urge

This book is a transcription and reproduction of the training course materials from Course #3 "Enable Your Life Urge"

The programming our subconscious mind gets from society is oriented towards us expecting to live short term lives and then dying in our seventies and eighties. It doesn't' have to be this way.

In this transcription of Course #3 of the 10 Principles of Personal Longevity, we learn how we have been programmed, and how we can change our subconscious mind towards a more positive outlook and a greater longevity view of life.

Longevity Training-Book 3 –Enable Your Life Urge

Longevity Training-Book 3 –Enable Your Life Urge

Copyright Page

The book is copyrighted for 2018

Longevity Training-Book 3-Enable Your Life Urge

By Martin K. Ettington

All Rights Reserved USA 2018

ISBN: 9781790935727

Printed in the United States of America

Longevity Training-Book 3 –Enable Your Life Urge

Longevity Training-Book 3 –Enable Your Life Urge

Other books by Martin K. Ettington

Spiritual and Metaphysics Books:
Prophecy: A History and How to Guide
God Like Powers and Abilities
Enlightenment for Newbies
Removing Illusions to Find True
        Happiness
Using the Scientific Method to Study
        the Paranormal
A Compendium of Metaphysics and
        How to Guides (Six books
        together in one volume)
Love from the Heart
The Enlightenment Experience
Learn Your Soul's Purpose
Pursuing Enlightenment
A Modern Man's Search for Truth
Use Intuition and Prophecy to Improve
        Your Life
The Handbook of Spiritual and Energy
        Healing

Longevity & Immortality:
Physical Immortality: A History and
        How to Guide
The Commentaries of Living Immortals
Records of Extremely Long Lived
        Persons
Enlightenment and Immortality
Longevity Improvements from Science
The 10 Principles of Personal
        Longevity
Telomeres & Longevity
The Diets and Lifestyles of the Worlds
        Oldest Peoples
The Longevity Six Books Bundle

Science Fiction:
Out of This Universe
Personal Freedom-Parts 1 & 2
The Psychic Soldier Series:
    Book 1-Himalayan Journey
    Book 2-A Soldier is Born
    Book 3-Fighting For Right
    Book 4-Earth Protector
The Immortality Sci Fi Bundle

The God Like Powers Series:
Human Invisibility
Invulnerability and Shielding
Teleportation
Psychokinesis
Our Energy Body, Auras, and
Thoughtforms

The God Like Powers Series—
        Volume 1 Compilation
The Yoga Discovery Series:
Yoga-An Ancient Art Form
Hatha Yoga-Helping you Live Better
Raja Yoga-Through the Ages
The Yoga Discovery Package

Business & Coaching Books:
Creating, Paublishing, & Marketing
        Practitioner Ebooks
Building a Successful Longevity
        Coaching Business
Why Become a Coach?
The Professional Coaching Success
Trilogy
2020-Make Money Writing and Selling
        Books
The 2020 Handbook of High Paying
        Work Without a College Degree

Science, Technology, and Misc.
Future Predictions By and Engineer &
        Seer
The Unusual Science & Technology
        Bundle
The Real Atlantis-In the Eye of the
        Sahara
Are Cryptozoological Animals Real or
        Imaginary?
Real Time Travel Stories From a
        Psychic Engineer
Removing Limits On Our
        Consciousness-And
        Thinking Outside the Box
33 Incredible True Survival Stories
How to Survive Anything: From the
        Wilderness to Man Made
        Disasters
All About Mars Journeys and
        Settlement
Mining the Asteroid Belt

Ancient History
The Real Atlantis-In the Eye of the
Sahara
Ancient & Prehistoric Civilizations
Ancient & Prehistoric Civilizations-Book
        Two
The History of Antediluvian Giants
The Antediluvian History of Earth
Ancient Underground Cities and
        Tunnels
Strange Objects Which Should Not Exist

Longevity Training-Book 3 –Enable Your Life Urge

Strange and Ancient Places in the USA
A Theory of Ancient Prehistory And
      Giant Aliens
<u>Aliens and Space</u>
Aliens and Secret Technology
Aliens Are Already Among Us
Designing and Building Space Colonies
Humanity and the Universe

All About Moon Bases
All About Mars Journeys and Settlement
The Space and Aliens Six Books Bundle
A Theory of Ancient Prehistory and
      Giant Aliens
The Space Colonies and Space
      Structures Coloring Book
All About Asteroids

<u>The Longevity Training Series</u>

(A transcription of the online Multimedia Longevity Coaching Training Program)

The Personal Longevity Training Series-Book1-Long Lived Persons
The Personal Longevity Training Series-Book2-Your Soul's Purpose
The Personal Longevity Training Series-Book3-Enable Your Life Urge
The Personal Longevity Training Series-Book4-Your Spiritual Connection
The Personal Longevity Training Series-Book5-Having Love in Your Heart
The Personal Longevity Training Series-Book6-Energy Body Health
The Personal Longevity Training Series-Book7-The Science of Longevity
The Personal Longevity Training Series-Book8-Physical Body Health
The Personal Longevity Training Series-Book9-Avoiding Accidents
The Personal Longevity Training Series-Book10-Implementing These Principles

The Personal Longevity Training Series-Books One Thru Ten

These books are all available in digital and printed formats from my
website and on Amazon, Barnes & Noble, Apple ITunes, and many other sites

My Books Website is: http://mkettingtonbooks.com

Longevity Training-Book 3 –Enable Your Life Urge

<u>Signup for our Mailing List to get the following:</u>

1) A discount coupon for 25% discount on all books on our site

2) Occasional Notices of new books available

3) Occasional Email on other offerings of ours (Monthly)

Go to this link to sign-up:

http://personal-longevity.com/mkebooks/emailsignup/

And click this link to get the FREE 102 page Ebook titled "Secrets of Many Things"

If you have any questions about this book or other subjects please contact the Author at:

mke@mkettingtonbooks.com

Table of Contents

Introduction

Back in 2008 I became very interested in the field of Longevity and Physical Immortality. After a lot of research this led me to my first book on the subject "Physical Immortality: A History and How to Guide". This book was pretty popular and I wanted to continue learning about Longevity and what things we could do about it in our lives.

The subject continued to fascinate me to the point that I developed a Longevity Coaching program over a couple of years starting in 2011. This online training program was multimedia—consisting of videos, my writings on longevity to read, online exercises, and tests for each of ten courses. It also included a lot of additional resources for each course including extra courses on how to become a successful Longevity Coach. A student who completed the training and tests successfully would become certified as a "Longevity Coach" and authorized to teach this material to others.

I developed a set of ten principles on longevity which are as follows:

The 10 Principles of Personal Longevity are:

- The Reality of Long Lived People
- Defining Your Purpose in Life
- Enabling the Life Urge
- Your Spiritual Health
- Having Love in Your Heart
- Energy Body Health
- The Science of Longevity
- Physical Body Health
- Using your Intuition for Safety
- Implementation of these principles

What are the 10 Principles all about?

The Reality of Long Lived People

The first principle is where I provide lots of evidence of people who have lived well over the age of 120 years old to 150-180-200, and even a 256 year old man from China:

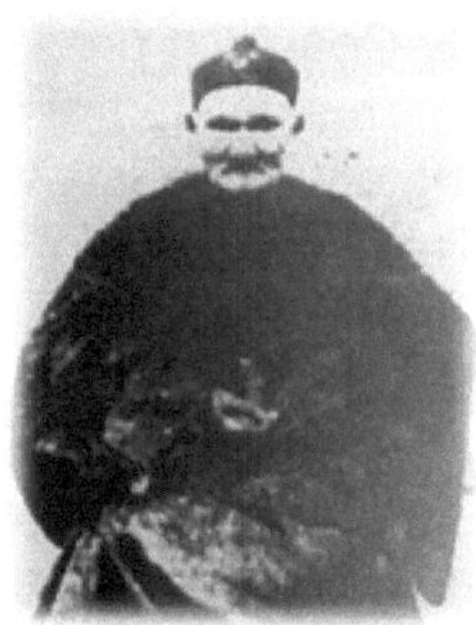

LI CHING-YUN: The Longest Lived person of record-256 Years (Source-The New York Times-May 6, 1933)

The Second Principle of Life Purpose

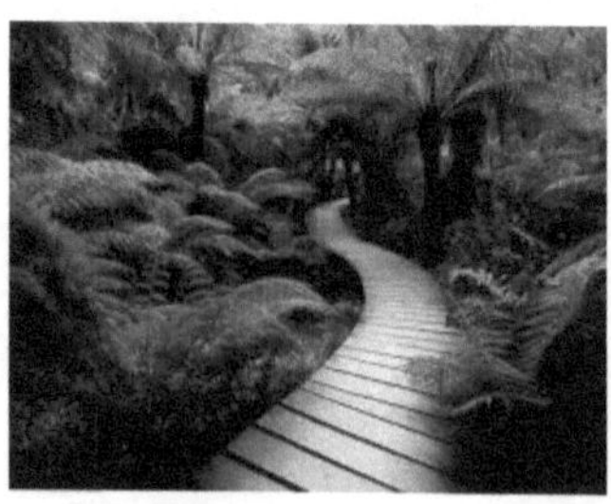

One of the things that occurred to me when I was putting the 10 principles together was that if one doesn't have a reason to live, or purpose in life--then what is the point?

This meant I had to add a very important step of how you can develop your own life purpose, or bring it up to date with your phase in life. Without reviewing your purpose-- then none of the rest of the principles matter.

Enabling the Life Urge

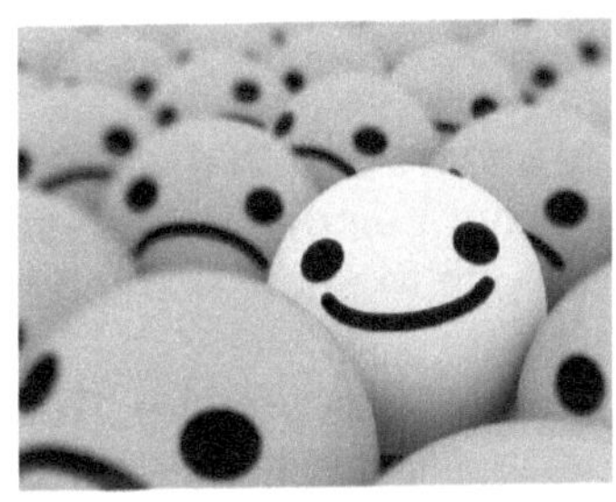

Have you ever realized how we are all programmed to expect to live through certain stages in life and then die? It's so common in our society that we don't think it odd that we expect to die at a certain age?

Have you ever heard radio ads saying "You are getting up in your sixties and seventies" so it's time to come out to our cemetery and buy a plot"

How ridiculous is this? And do you see how much our subconscious has been programmed towards death?

This principle is all about reprogramming ourselves to have a more positive outlook on life and its possibilities.

Having a Spiritual Connection in Your Life

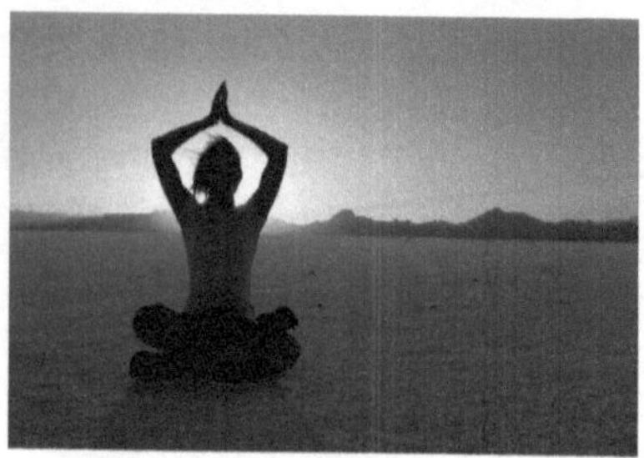

Most of us innately understand that we have a spiritual core in the center of our being. It is this spiritual core that we need to connect with to enable our physical health too.

It doesn't matter what religion you are. Regular meditation, deep prayer, or just walking in the woods helps you make and keep that connection in your life.

Having Love in Your Heart

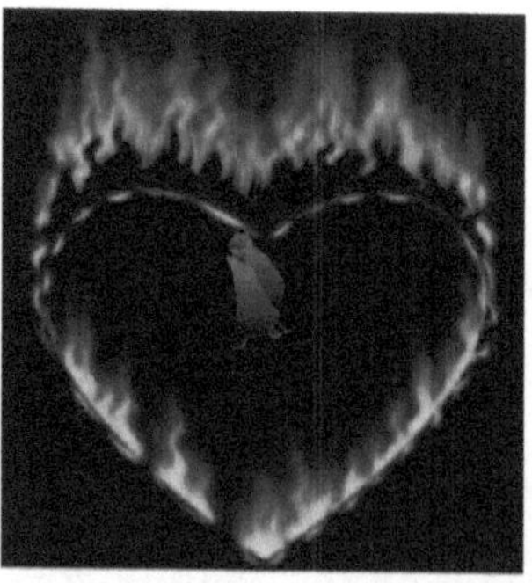

One of the most important things I learned in the last five years was that Unconditional Love is a real and physical thing. It is a powerful energy force in life and not just a philosophical belief system.

I considered it so important that I added it as a separate principle of longevity.

True Unconditional Love is healing, embodies happiness, and is a powerful part of our vital forces.

Energy Body Health

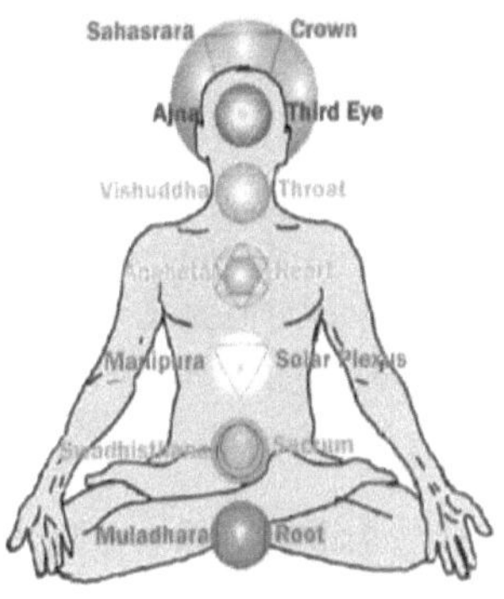

We all have an energy body which is part of our vital forces. The Indians talk about the "Chakras" and the Chinese talk about "Energy Meridians" in Acupuncture.

We should all learn different practices to keep our vital forces flowing for maximum health and vitality.

The Science of Longevity

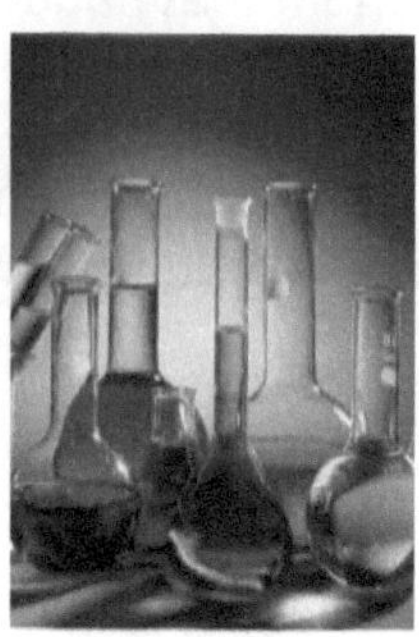

Science and Medicine are making new discoveries all the time that we can take advantage of to extend our lives. Why not take advantage of these discoveries which provide new therapies and supplements to increase our longevity.

There is also a lot we can learn from plants and animals. We all share the same genetic basis.

Some of these plants and animals live thousands of years and some cells are immortal.

What can we learn from them to apply to our lives?

Physical Body Health

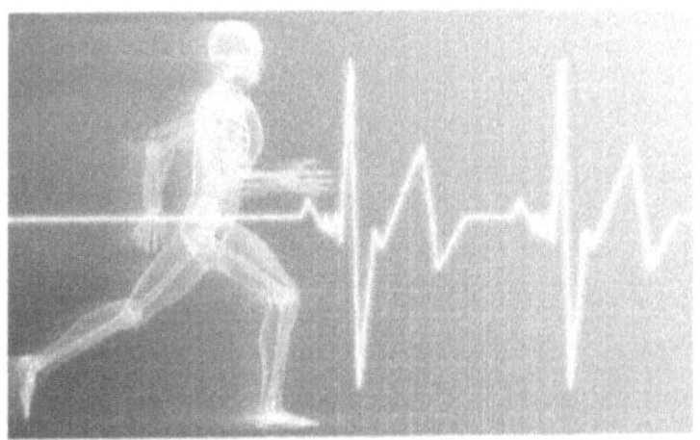

There are many types of supplements used for anti-aging for thousands of years. What can we learn about them that we can apply to our lives?

What other considerations about our physical health does nontraditional or alternative medicine offer?

Using Your Intuition for Safety

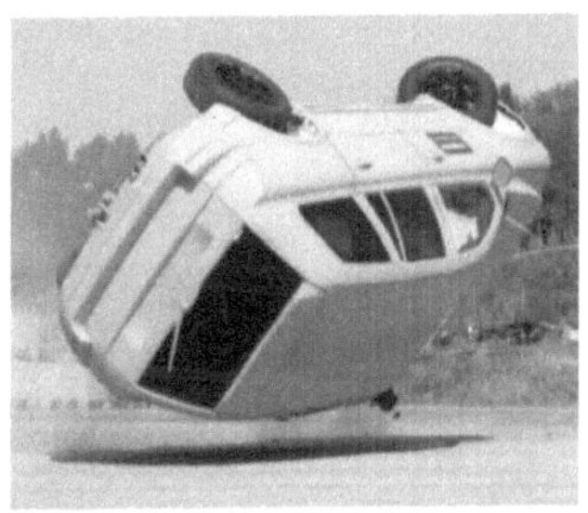

Once you have established your own long term health then what is the greatest danger you face?

ACCIDENTS

We can learn to use our intuition to make us safer as well as see potential future events which may be good too.

Why not open up to the possibilities of how our spirit has this natural ability in all of us?

Implementing These Principles in Your Life

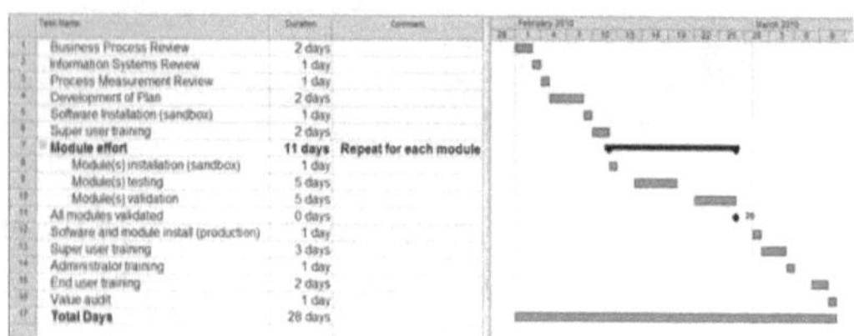

It's nice to read about all these concepts, but how can you really apply them to your own life?

This is what the chapter on implementation is all about, and it helps you plan a lifelong change in your health focus to live these principles and truly experience long term health, greater happiness, and extended longevity.

For five years I amended and improved these materials which now include a lot more information and helpful concepts for students wanting to improve their longevity and those of others.

I transcribed my videos and other materials to this book so you can read it all, and later hear it in an AudioBook.

This book is priced pretty inexpensively, compared to the online training and certification program which sells in total for $1,995 USD. If you are interested in taking the entire online program at a major discount, then please contact me at:

Marty@personal-longevity.com

Hope you enjoy these materials since when applied correctly they will significantly change your life.

PLP Concepts Overview

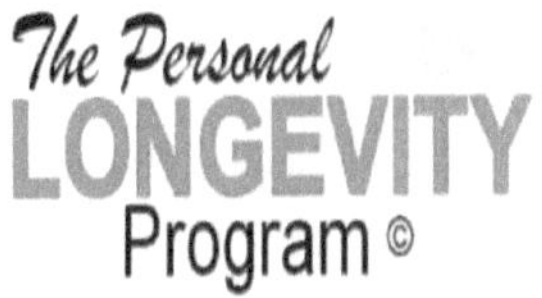

(Transcription of overview video)

Hello I'm Martin Ettington and I'd like to introduce you to the Personal Longevity Program which is an integrated holistic approach to long-term health. In this video we will only cover the high level concepts which comprise individual courses in the coaching certificate program for personal longevity.

The first concept is that long lived people exist and have existed for hundreds of thousands of years. We cover in the first course all about their records; along with people not only in places you might think like India, but in Europe and the United States-people who've lived long lives and well documented cases.

We discuss people who have lived well over the age of 120 and even the case of a Chinaman who lived to 256 years old. Plus a lot of mythology about people who have lived even longer lives so you get an idea that extending your life much longer than we think is currently medically and scientifically possible is certainly something that can happen.

The second course's concept has to do with finding your souls purpose. The point of wanting to live a long life is to know what your purpose in life is, so we go through some readings and some exercises to help you determine where soul's purpose in life is. Then doing goals as a fundamental concept so you will know the motivations in your life.

Third is the "Psychology of Living" also known by certain practitioners as "Removing the death Urge". The psychology of living has to do with seeking a positive image about your ability to live a long time. We tend to be programmed from birth about the idea that we are going to go through certain stages in our life as a child, as a teenager, and as adults. It's about reprogramming your subconscious as to the possibilities of a long life.

I've also learned in my life that it is very important to be able open your heart to unconditional love. When you're able to love unconditionally it also helps increase the strength of your immune system and fight off disease. So this is an aspect of spiritual growth. The courses also cover unconditional love and energy body forces. Managing your energy body is an important component of who you are in having energy working properly in your body and is another aspect of health for the length of longevity.

There are many types of scientific and medical research which are being done today and which will contribute to human longevity in the future.

Do you know that the average lifespan in the United States in 1900 was only about 40 years? We have doubled lifespan in the last century with current technologies but things under way in terms of scientific and medical improvements will help extend your lives further.

Also in this course on longevity we will cover a lot of the concepts which are being researched by scientists today. There are suggestions for more things you can do to do to use this science to improve your health along with physical supplements.

A unique thing that I thought about and decided to offer in these courses has to do with all my experiences in prophecy and how I was able to change outcomes on accidents that would occur to me by using simple exercises you can learn to change these outcomes. If you're in great health often the biggest thing you have to worry about are accidents.

We also provide guidelines you can follow on a daily basis and plans you can make to live healthier and happier and have a much longer life than you ever thought possible.

Thank you for listening !

Course #3 Intro Video

(Transcription of Video)

Hi! This is Marty Ettington and I'd like to welcome you to the Personal Longevity Program. This is course number three on the psychology of living. What is the Psychology of Living? Also known as "Removing the Death Urge".

This is all about the subconscious beliefs about our lives- how long we can live? And what are the limiting beliefs about what we can do to lengthen our lives?
In other words, how are we programmed birth?

We are typically programmed from birth to expect to live different phases of our life. We are going to be a baby, a child, a teenager, an adult, and then we are going to die after a certain period of time. This is programmed into our lives.

Also, you may have heard some advertising that "You're getting up there into your sixties and seventies. Why not come into our cemetery and buy a plot? Cause now it's getting close to time" You are being programmed to expect to die.

Or have you ever met an old couple—I have—who was very healthy in their eighties and then one of them died. And the other one over six months lost weight, got sick, and died; because this woman lost her will to live.

So the will to live, to want to live a long life is a very important part of the psychology of living. So in this course we are going to work on turning the death urge into a life urge. We are going to talk about books to read and videos to watch which have inspiration. How to be inspired—like this beautiful background behind me. The rocks, flow of water, and beautiful plants which inspired you to love the world again.

Or for instance, have you ever seen a painting, or building, or new technology industry which gets you to say "Wow this incredible" These are things that inspire you.

Through a series of inspirational writings and affirmations we are going to work on trying to change your "Death Urge" into a "Life Urge". The exercises in this course will be used to do this too.

Enabling Your Life Urge

From the Book "The 10 Principles of Personal Longevity"

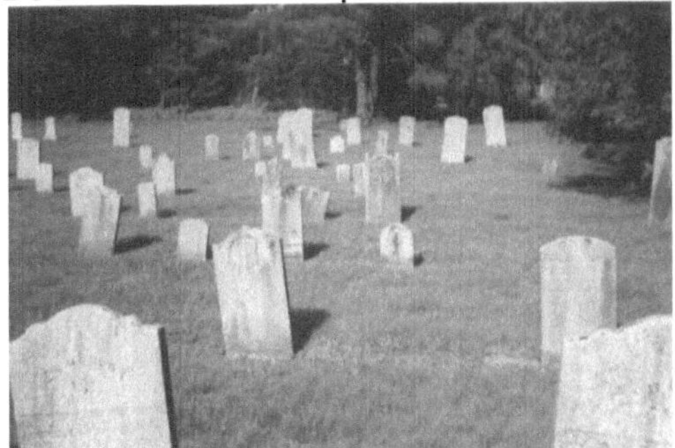

The Third Principle of personal longevity is about changing the subconscious programming we all learn from birth in our society.

This programming is that we are expected to go through certain stages in life and then die.

An example from my life:

I had a paper route when I was eleven years old and one of my customers was an old couple in their eighties—family friends named the Burrus.

They were very healthy until the man died one day—I don't know from what. After that his wife got thinner and thinner each week that I saw her until she just died after six more months because she had no more will to live.

She had decided it was her time to die. How many of us have known persons like this who just gave up and quit? You have to want to live and long time and know that you can do it to make it possible in your life.

We can change our programming to know deep down that we are able to live much longer and have more fulfilling lives than we ever thought possible.

Leonard Orr:

Much of the wisdom on the life urge is from the teachings of Leonard Orr. Leonard is an unconventional thinker of the 1960s and 1970s.

He started the re-birthing movement in San Francisco during the 1960's New Age era in San Francisco. He also wrote a book called "Breaking the Death Habit" which is now out of print but can be obtained at my website http://mkettingtonbooks.com

In this book he says that he met many immortals in India and the Himalayas who were all at least 300 years old or more.

He learned a lot of his knowledge from an ascended master "Babaji" who has been around for thousands of years.

He says that disciples first need to work on developing a philosophy of physical immortality.

Leonard says: "The physiology of physical immortality is based on inner awareness of our energy body. One must learn how to clean and balance the energy body on a daily basis with earth, air, water, and fire.

Second you need to unravel the "Death Urge" which is built into all family traditions through the psychology of physical immortality. By this Leonard means the expectation built

into almost everyone's subconscious that we will all live an average life span, and then die.
Here are some of the death urges built into our subconscious which we learn growing up in our civilization:

The belief that we will physically slow down starting in our thirties, become much less mobile in our sixties and bedridden in our eighties

The image we project on older people that they aren't as attractive or healthy as younger people—this image affects them too

Advertising to start planning for your own funeral

Retirement Planning only looking at a timeframe of living into your eighties—because you will not need any money after that Social Security and Medicare—we will not be able to take care of ourselves when we retire

The belief that the mind will lose its memory and ability to think clearly as it ages
That old people are ugly

That there will be nothing interesting to do after kids move away and we retire from our job

That old people need to make space in society for the young

Medical care being reduced for old people, and sometimes withheld—because they will die anyway

The third step is the mastery of the physical body. This can be accomplished by certain breathing exercises and practices.

The final step is where spiritual purification exercises come in.

We recommend people start by saying the following to themselves every day:

"My life urges are strong, in control, and keep me continuously alive and in perfect robust health.

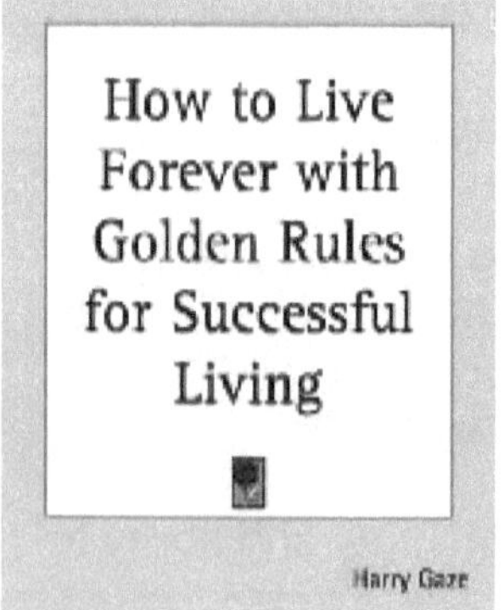

The following book by Harry Gaze in an excellent source of re-programing and positive thinking to help us change our programming about how long we believe we can live.

Golden Rules to Live Forever

Harry Gaze was a Philosopher and Teacher back in the early 20th Century. He was a teacher and lecturer in practical Metaphysics, New Thought, and Divine Science. He began his lecture work as early as 1898 and published numerous books on Metaphysics.

His book titled "How to Live Forever with Golden Rules for Successful Living" is very relevant to our study of physical immortality, and was first published in 1905. (He also wrote an earlier work on the subject in 1904 titled "How to Live Forever, The Science and Practice").

Like some other writers on the subject of unlimited longevity he believed that growing old and the body decaying was not inevitable! His belief was that the power of the spirit and thought on the body could keep one young forever.

Harry believed in several principles which guided his thinking:

The body literally and completely returns to dust in less than one year, and during this period, a new body is constructed molecule by molecule.

Conscious cooperation with this change is the secret to eternal youth.

Old age and somatic death are brought about by conditions which can be   effectually prevented.

He had a set of Golden Rules for Eternal Youth which are reproduced here:

Golden Rule for Eternal Youth Number One: Realize there is one divine life in which you live, move, and have your being.

Golden Rule for Eternal Youth Number Two: Realize that as a Son of God you are heir to God's immortality here and now; claim your birthright.

Golden Rule for Eternal Youth Number Three: Realize that your body is a template of the Holy Spirit.

Golden Rule for Eternal Youth Number Four: Deeply realize that your body is an expression of your mind, and attune yourself to infinite spirit.

Golden Rule for Eternal Youth Number Five: Realize that by virtue of molecular renewal, which is constantly in operation, your body is constantly made new.

Golden Rule for Eternal Youth Number Six: Keep in mind that nature's constant renewal of the body gives the opportunity of building a better body with each succeeding renewal.

Golden Rule for Eternal Youth Number Seven: Practice rhythmical breathing and freely use your diaphragm, the organ that is the muscular   floor of your upper internal organs, and the ceiling of your lower organs.

Golden Rule for Eternal Youth Number Eight: Realize that eternal youth is harmony and positive cooperation with the upward law of continuous growth and the law of attraction.

Golden Rule for Eternal Youth Number Nine: Realize that the secret of eternal youth is cooperation with God in creative, individual, volitional evolution.

Golden Rule for Eternal Youth Number Ten: Practice faithfully the daily affirmations for Eternal Youth, doing them in a regular, cumulative   sequence.

Golden Rule for Eternal Youth Number Eleven: Practice concentrative exercises daily, and develop control of attention and thought selectivity. Also do meditative exercises and the Silence.

(Note the focus on meditation in Rule Eleven. This was a very unusual term to use one hundred years ago and indicates some familiarity with knowledge from the East.)

Golden Rule for Eternal Youth Number Twelve: Realize the oneness of your inner Christ life with God, thinking of God as an Infinite Life, Infinite Power, Infinite Health, Infinite Youth, Infinite Peace, Infinite Joy.

Rule number 10 mentions the daily affirmations for Eternal Youth. These are listed below too. Mr. Gaze recommends practicing one daily for the whole month, then starting over again:

Adaptation: Whenever essential, I adapt myself readily to more perfect change.

Adjustment: I give myself freely to wise, spiritual, mental, and physical adjustment.

Beauty: I realize that the beauty of enduring youth is as deep as the innermost recesses of the soul.

Buoyancy: In every thought, nerve, and muscle I express the perfect buoyancy of joyous youth.

Confidence: I cheerfully react to all conditions with the boundless   confidence of youth.

Courage: I increasingly attain the natural courage of strong and vital youth.

Creativeness: The Divine Spirit, everywhere, and in and through me, inspires me with keen creativeness.
Daring: I blend the pure daring of youth with the wisdom of growth and experience.

Elasticity: My sense of freedom and flexibility of mind find its correspondence in bodily elasticity.

Energy: My whole being is vitally energized with the radiant life of the Divine Spirit.

Flexibility: I joyously affirm the quality of flexibility in every cell, muscle and artery of my being.

Freshness: Bathing in the commonness of pure spirit, I am fresh as the dawn of day.

Gracefulness: By wise exercise, relaxation, visualization and nourishment, I maintain the gracefulness of youth.

Happiness: I realize that the true spring of happiness is within me.

Initiative: The spirit of initiative and wise adventure freely motivates and activates me.
Joy: The joy of eternal youth is my daily light and inspiration.

Loveliness: The loveliness of ever-renewing youth is the expression of loving and lovable qualities.

Newness: Every day and every moment, my body is being made new in every cell, molecule and atom.

Optimism: I look joyously forward with the spirit of youthful optimism.

Progressiveness: I am a progressive conscious, purposeful and individual factor in my evolution.

Purity: I see life with the eyes of childlike purity blended with power and poise.

Radiance: I am radiant with the light, life and love of infinite wisdom.

Receptivity: Knowing that I am a child of God, I am at all times receptive to the highest inspiration.

Rejuvenation: I am devoted and consecrated to all habits that rejuvenate   and heal.

Renewal: I am an ever-renewing and ever-unfolding expression of infinite life.

Responsiveness: As the years unfold, I maintain my full, free responsiveness to the best in life.

Unfoldment: I am open, receptive and responsive to new growth and unfoldments.

Versatility: I joyously express the creative spirit in me in the versatility that unites youth with experience.

Vitality: I think, speak, breathe, exercise, relax and nourish my mind and   body for increasing vitality.

Youth: I realize that the fountain of Eternal Youth, like the Kingdom of God, is here and now, within me.

Zest: My thought, speech and action are all radiantly animated with youthful zest for living.

A Positive Outlook on Life

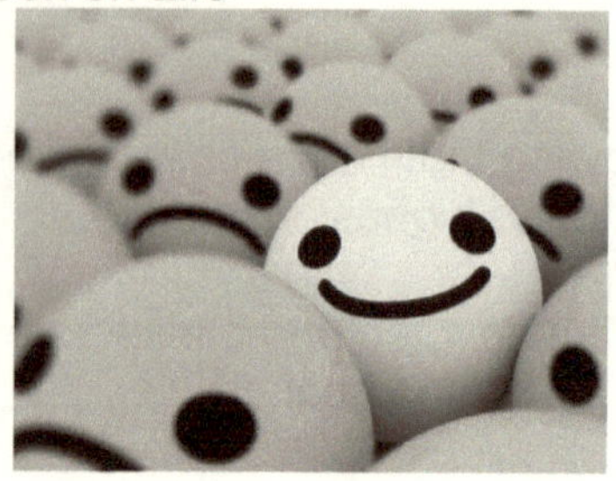

How does a positive outlook on life increase your life span?

Optimism and a positive outlook increases our vitality and spiritual connections.

If you are positive you have a better chance of extracting yourself from an unhealthful or dangerous situation.

An article extract from an M.D. reinforces the importance of a positive outlook:

"Optimism is necessary for good health," says Charles L. Raison, MD, a psychiatrist and director of the behavioral immunology clinic at Emory University School of Medicine in Atlanta. "There's growing evidence that, for many medical illnesses, stress and a negative mental state -- pessimism, feeling overwhelmed, being burnt out -- has a negative effect on immunity, which is especially important in rheumatoid arthritis."

Indeed, your brain can create all sorts of tailor-made prescriptions to nurture your body. Raison says these include endorphins -- the natural painkillers; gamma globulin, which fortifies your immune system; and interferon, which helps combat infections, viruses, even cancer.

When depression sets in, we're less likely to take care of ourselves, which means the brain doesn't get prompted to produce those great natural remedies, Raison says. We don't exercise, because we don't have much energy. We don't eat right. We lose sleep -- or we sleep too much.

Visualizing your Immortal Future

Here is an exercise to help you see yourself alive far into the future…

The key to visualizing your physically immortal future is not to imagine that you will get there but to imagine that you are already there. The more vividly you can imagine being immortal now and what you are doing very vividly, the more this changes the probability of your future to make it so.

Here is an excellent exercise to help you visualize yourself in health and happiness in your own immortal future:

Relax for 5-10 minutes.

Choose a happy scene of family, friends, or profession or activities   that you want to visualize.

We are going to picture the scene you have chosen at different ages. These ages will be 100, 200, and 500 years old. As you visualize you will be in that scene. You make it real. You will put energy and will into it to   make it happen.

You are now 100 years old. You are in the scene. People and scenery are around you. You can feel the temperature; the light in the sky or   ceiling. You also smell the scene and you see everything vividly. You can look around and see details such as trees or on buildings or walls, etc.

Your body feels healthy and you can tell you are youthful. Your solid belief in your own immortality has been paying off for a while now.

You are now 200 years old and it's the 23rd century. (Your lifestyle may have changed to something which is an earlier period in a place where change is slower). Again, see your surroundings very vividly in a scene you enjoy. Feel all five senses.

What do you see?
What do you hear?
What do you smell?
What do you taste?
What do you feel?

You are now 500 years old and it's the 25th century. You may have travelled out into the solar system or to a planet around another star. Life goes on and you are in a community of other immortals who have similar interests to you.

Maybe you are getting educated for a new profession, or maybe you are an artist in a mode you never tried before. You have probably learned to teleport yourself by this time and live totally in the now. Look around you to see what's there. You feel very strong and healthy as you usually do, and you have now been healthy and physically stable for centuries.

Keep doing this imagery consistently every day for a few minutes until you start to feel solidity and that the events will happen. This is when you now that your will and energy have created the future.

You might want to record this visualization on tape to play back to yourself. Your own voice is the most powerful voice you can hear.

The Big Book of Inspiring Stories

Foreword

This volume features a selection of the world's most inspiring stories to move the body and soul. Inspire your readers with these tales of courage and bravery so that they can have a breakthrough in their own struggles, no matter where they are. Featured in this massive book are tales of people overcoming extraordinary hardship and achieving breakthroughs in their lives. Their strength and courage serve as a source of inspiration and motivation for us all.

The Big Book of Inspiring Stories -A Powerful Collection of Tales of Courage that Inspires and Strengthens the Soul

Chapter 1: Success Stories of Great People

Success Stories of Great People and Inspiring Leaders

Thomas Alva Edison is one of America's most famous inventors. Edison saw huge change take place in his lifetime. He was responsible for making many of those changes occur. His inventions created and contributed to modern night lights, movies, telephones, records and CDs. Edison was truly a genius. Edison is most famous for his development of the first electric light bulb. When Edison was born, electricity had not been developed. By the time he died, entire cities were lit by electricity. Much of the credit for electricity goes to Edison. Some of his inventions were improvements on other inventions, like the telephone. Some of his inventions he deliberately tried to invent, like the light bulb and the movie projector. But some inventions he stumbled upon, like the phonograph. Of all his inventions, Edison was most proud of the phonograph.

Edison invented and improved upon things that transformed our world. Some things he invented by himself. Some things he invented with other people. Just about all his inventions are things we still use in some form today. Throughout his life, Edison tried to invent things that everyone could use.

Edison created the world's first "invention factory". He and his partners invented, built and shipped the product - all in the same complex. This was a new way to do business. Today many businesses have copied Edison's invention factory design. A business friend once asked Edison about the secret to his success. Edison replied, "Genius is hard work, stick-to-itiveness, and common sense". But his "common sense" was very uncommon. More patents were issued to Edison than have been issued to any other single person in U.S. history: 1,093.

Beethoven was born on 16th, December, 1770 in Bonn of Germany. His father was a singer in local palace choir. Beethoven's father was a very common person and he was addicted to gambling. However, his mother was a fairly kind-hearted and gentle female. She married an assistant as her first marriage and married to Beethoven's father when her ex-husband died. Beethoven didn't have access to go to school for the reason that his family was very poor. Nevertheless, he had a special feeling of music when he was very young. His father wanted to make use of his potential to make a big fortune. As a result, Beethoven had to practice playing clavicorn and violin day and night under his father's pressure.

Beethoven had a performance on a stage for the first time when he was only seven years old and he made a huge success. Some famous musicians considered him as the second Mozart. Beethoven learned how to compose music from Nifo and published his first work named Concerto in A minor when he was 11. He went to Vienna to learn how to compose music from Mozart and Haydn. It seems that he would have a fairly bright future when Beethoven received the first success in 1800. Nevertheless, he was troubled with a terrible matter for years at that time. He found that he has become a deaf person. There couldn't be anything more terrible than that for a musician. He sank into a blue mood for a long time as a consequence.

Beethoven has an enthusiastic heart all the time. But his enthusiasm was often unfortunate. He often tolerated both hope and enthusiasm, disappointment and resistance. There was no doubt that all of these emotions had become his unique source of creation. He fell in love with Julia in 1801 and composed a music named Moonlight for her specifically. To his disappointed, she couldn't understand his noble soul and refused him. Beethoven was upset and despairing for that and married before long. It was the most hopeless moment for him and once a time, he wrote down a paper of posthumous papers.

He came to life in 1803 and composed some bright and warm music such as The Second Symphonies. From then on, several more beautiful and marvelous music were produced. Some of them are fairly famous and I think you must have heard about them such as The Eroica and The Storm. Beethoven finished his masterpiece named The Ninth Symphonies in 1823. This piece of work expressed his world in his dream. He suffered from pulmonary edema in Dec.1826, which was resulted from a bad influenza. He passed away on 26th, March, 1827 for the reason of suffering from hepatopathy.

It is said that the day on which Beethoven died was raining heavily and storming seriously. It seems that even the God grieved over his death. Beethoven's funeral was fairly solemn and grand. It is estimated that over 20 thousand people presented his funeral.

Mother Teresa - This great personality was born in Albania. Right from the age of 18, Agnes Gonxha Bojaxhiu, popularly known as mother Teresa, was into spirituality. It was in the year 1931, when this young girl with a golden heart, acquired the name Teresa from the French nun Thérèse Martin. In 1937, she took vows and began teaching in Saint Mary's High School in Calcutta. In 1948, she got another opportunity from God to serve the society. The same year, mother Teresa was relieved by

Pope Pious XII from her services and she was granted the status of an independent nun. And thereafter, she got engrossed with the task of serving the poor and sick people of Calcutta. The coming years witnessed the setting up of a charity organization called the Missionaries of Charity. In 1950, her source of concern was the care of lepers, the people discarded by society.

Missionary of Charity opened its branches in almost every country to assist the poor, elderly, blind and people suffering from deadly disease like AIDS. For the bright future of children, she opened up schools. In 1979, she was awarded with Nobel Prize for the services that she had rendered to the society. But the journey of this great messiah on earth ended in August 1997, when she made her way towards the heaven.

Michael Jordan is one of the greatest basketball players of all time. Although, a summary of his basketball career and influence on the game inevitably fails to do it justice, as a phenomenal athlete with a unique combination of fundamental soundness, grace, speed, power, artistry, improvisational ability and an unquenchable competitive desire, Jordan single-handedly redefined the NBA superstar.

Even contemporaneous superstars recognized the unparalleled position of Jordan. Magic Johnson said, "There's Michael Jordan and then there is the rest of us." Larry Bird, following a playoff game where Jordan dropped 63 points on the Boston Celtics in just his second season, appraisal of the young player was: "God disguised as Michael Jordan."

A brief listing of his top accomplishments would include the following: Rookie of the Year; Five-time NBA MVP; Six-time NBA champion; Six-time NBA Finals MVP; Ten-time All-NBA First Team; Nine time NBA All-Defensive First Team; Defensive Player of the Year; 14-time NBA All-Star; Three-time NBA All-Star MVP; 50th Anniversary All-Time Team; Ten scoring titles -- an NBA record and seven consecutive matching Wilt Chamberlain; Retired with the NBA's highest scoring average of 30.1ppg.

Michael Jordan makes the jump shot that catapults the Bulls over the Utah Jazz in the 1998 Finals. However, his impact is far greater than awards and championships. He burst into the league as a rookie sensation scoring in droves with an unmatchable first step and acrobatic drives and dunks and concluded his career as a cultural Icon. Along the way, he became a true champion who spearheaded the globalization of the NBA with his dynamic on court abilities and personal sense of style that was marketed to the masses.

He was an accessible star who managed to maintain an air of mystique. He was visible as "Air Jordan," as part of a sneaker advertising campaign and endorsing other products as well as the star of the movie, Space Jam. However, he would vanish into retirement twice only to return until hanging up the sneakers for the last time after the 2002-03 season. Although Brooklyn born, Jordan was bred in the more tranquil North Carolina. The son of Delores and James Jordan, he shared a special bond with his father, which included baseball being both of their first love. However, following his older brother, Larry, whom he idolized and was a spectacular athlete in his own right, Jordan began to play basketball. Jordan, coming off a gold medal performance at the 1984 Olympics prospered in the pro game with a fabulous first season, earning the NBA Rookie of the Year Award. He averaged 28.2 ppg, (third behind Bernard King and Bird) 6.5 rpg and 5.9 apg. He also was selected to the All-NBA Second Team. Perhaps more important, the Bulls improved to win 11 more games than in the season prior to his arrival and made it to the playoffs. Jordan averaged 29.3 ppg in the first round series, but the Bulls lost in four games to the Milwaukee Bucks.

In his first season, he did not have outstanding shooting range and was thought to roam to often on defense resulting from playing trapping defenses in college according to his first NBA coach, Kevin Loughery. Yet, his medium game -- eight to 15-feet from the basket was impressive as evidenced by his .515 field-goal shooting percentage and his steals tended to compensate for his less than stellar straight-up defense. Improvement in both areas would come and he would ultimately be regarded as threat from anywhere on the floor and one of the best ever one-on-one defenders.

"There's Michael Jordan and then there is the rest of us." -- Magic Johnson Even in the exhibition season before his rookie campaign, players and coaches were sure that the Rockets and Blazers would regret their picks. King, the eventual leading scorer for that upcoming season, seemed sure as well when he spoke to Hoop magazine after a 1984 preseason game. "All I can say," King says, "is that the people in Chicago are in for a real treat." He was right. Jordan's greatness and likeabilty was apparent in just his first season. Home attendance at the venerable Chicago Stadium and on the road rose dramatically. Fans of opposing teams were seemingly content to see their team lose if in return Jordan put on a show. Jordan's personal style was equally authentic and unique as his basketball skills. Nike signed him to a major shoe deal because of his anticipated appeal, but he surpassed even the loftiest of expectations.

One version of the sneakers he wore in his first preseason was an unseen before blend of his team's red and black colors that the NBA initially considered in violation of the "uniformity of uniform rule." Subject to fines if he continued to wear them, he occasionally did and the demand for that version and others in the Air Jordan line was unprecedented.

The rookie's mesmerizing effect was even suggested to have extended to referees as it was said that he was getting veteran preferential treatment allowing him to take that additional step on route to the basket rather than being whistle for a travelling violation. Many assessed that he eluded defenders so easily that he had to be travelling. However, video break down established that his first step was just so quick and that he was not in violation of the rulebook. Despite all the attention, Jordan retained a sense of humility. He did not ridicule the Blazers for not taking him. Early on in his first season, he told Sports Illustrated, "He [Bowie] fits in better than I would. They have an overabundance of big guards and small forwards." His self-effacement was more apparent when in that same article he said, "I'd like to play in at least one All-Star game." Three games into his second season, he broke a bone in his left foot. He was voted to the All-Star team but could not play as he was sidelined for 64 games. However, he came back late in the year to score a NBA playoff-record 63 points in a first-round game against the Celtics. The Bulls lost that game 132-131 in double-overtime and the series in a sweep, but Jordan averaged 43.7 ppg in the series. If there were any doubters to that point about Jordan's ability, surely there were no more.

The success story behind Berkshire Hathaway's Warren Buffett---who is also the company's largest shareholder and CEO---spans back to his years packing groceries at his grandfather's grocery store. Buffet showed maturity beyond his years when he decided that he would rather make money than play games with the other children his age.

Born Warren Edward Buffett on August 30, 1930 to a stock broker turned-Congressman, it is no wonder that Buffett showed an amazing flair for business and numbers at such an early age. At 11 years old, he jumped into the world of high finance by buying three shares of Cities Service that he later sold. He immediate regretted the decision as the numbers for Cities Service soared. Buffett learned his lessons earlier than most, paving the way for the plethora of critical real-world decisions he was going to make. Warren Buffett was educated at Woodrow Wilson High School, Washington, D.C. after his father was elected into Congress. He received his college education at The Wharton School, University of Pennsylvania then later at the University of Nebraska where he received a B.S. in Economics. Choosing to further his education, Buffett enrolled at the Columbia Business School where he graduated in 1951 with an M.S. in Economics.

Warren Buffett experienced a variety of jobs before he landed himself at Berkshire Hathaway. Fresh out of school, he worked as an investment salesman at Buffett-Falk & Co., Omaha until 1954. From 1954 to 1956, Buffett served at Graham-Newman Corp., New York as a Securities Analyst. from 1956-1969, he sat as a General Partner at the Buffett Partnership, Ltd. Since 1970, Buffet has served at Berkshire Hathaway Inc., Omaha as its Chairman and CEO. Berkshire Hathaway Inc. is a conglomerate holding company that oversees and manages a number of subsidiary companies. Since coming onboard, Buffet has been instrumental in driving the company to the colossal status it stands at today. In 2008, Warren Buffet was ranked number one on Forbes list of World's Billionaires making this the richest success story in the world.

Bill Gates was born on October 28, 1955 in a family having rich business, political and community service background. His great-grandfather was a state legislator and a mayor, his grandfather was vice president of national bank and his father was a lawyer. Bill strongly believes in hard work. He believes that if you are intelligent and know how to apply your intelligence, you can achieve anything. From childhood Bill was ambitious, intelligent and competitive. These qualities helped him to attain top position in the profession he chose. In school, he had an excellent record in mathematics and science. Still he was getting very bored in school and his parents knew it, so they always tried to feed him with more information to keep him busy. Bill's parents came to know their son's intelligence and decided to enroll him in a private school, known for its intense academic environment. It was a very important decision in Bill Gate's life where he was first introduced to a computer. Bill Gates and his friends were very much interested in computer and formed "Programmers Group" in late 1968. Being in this group, they found a new way to apply their computer skill in University of Washington. In the next year, they got their first opportunity in Information Sciences Inc. in which they were selected as programmers. ISI (Information Sciences Inc.) agreed to give them royalties whenever it made money from any of the group's program. As a result of the business deal signed with Information Sciences Inc., the group also became a legal business.

Bill Gates and his close friend Allen started new company of their own, Traf-O-Data. They developed a small computer to measure traffic flow. From this project they earned around $20,000. The era of Traf-O-Data came to an end when Gates left the college. In 1973, he left home for Harvard University. He didn't know what to do, so he enrolled his name for pre-law. He took the standard freshman courses with the exception of signing up for one of Harvard's toughest mathematics courses. He did well over there, but he couldn't find it interesting too. He spent many long nights in front of the school's computer and the next day asleep in class. After leaving school, he almost lost himself from the world of computers. Gates and his friend Paul Allen remained in close contact even though they were away from school. They would often discuss new ideas for future projects and the possibility of starting a business one fine day. At the end of Bill's first year, Allen came close to him so that they could follow some of their ideas. That summer they got job in Honeywell. Allen kept on pushing Bill for opening a new software company. Within a year, Bill Gates dropped out from Harvard. Then he formed Microsoft. Microsoft's vision is "A computer on every desk and Microsoft software on every computer". Bill is a visionary person and works very hard to achieve his vision. His belief in high intelligence and hard work has put him where he is today. He does not believe in mere luck or God's grace, but just hard work and competitiveness. Bill's Microsoft is good competition for other software companies and he will continue to stomp out the competition until he dies. He likes to play the game of Risk and the game of world domination. His beliefs are so powerful, which have helped him increase his wealth and his monopoly in the industry.

Bill Gates is not a greedy person. In fact, he is quite giving person when it comes to computers, internet and any kind of funding. Some years back, he visited Chicago's Einstein Elementary School and announced grants benefiting Chicago's schools and museums where he donated a total of $110,000, a bunch of computers, and provided internet connectivity to number of schools. Secondly, Bill Gates donated 38 million dollars for the building of a computer institute at Stanford University. Gates plans to give away 95% of all his earnings when he is old and gray. Bill Gates from this story may seem a superhero and do it alone guy but in reality, he is not. He was able to achieve it because of the kind of people that he choose to mingle with.

Chapter 2: Overcoming Adversity

Oprah Winfrey - No one ever blames Oprah Winfrey for taking some easy way out. Although her childhood was full of toil, this young girl from Kosciusko, Mississippi always believed she was destined to be someone great.

Maybe it was from her life background in a village that she learned "to turn misery into wisdom" as she stated later. And her misery was not just a few. She was born as she resulted of a free intercourse between her mother and a service man who then left her. First Oprah was brought up by her grandmother in a pig farm with no running water facility. She then lived with her mother who moved to Milwaukee where she was sexually abused for the first time by a friend of her family and her own relative. Oprah grew up into a rebellious teenager, at 14 years old she lived in a bad surroundings and gave birth to a male baby that died a week later. Losing her patience, Oprah's Mother sent her to live with her father – a man she never knew before.

But it was by living with her father that she eventually got the discipline she needed to turn her outstanding intelligence into its right track. She was doing well at school and was known for her smart talking. She joined a local beauty contest and won a scholarship in Tennessee State University. She began to study broadcast communication and got a part time job as a reporter in Nashville TV station.

Suddenly it looked like nothing could ever stop the strides of this young girl who was once was a naughty girl. Oprah left school at the age as young as 19 years old to become the first Afro-American woman broadcaster in Nashville. She wrestled with this job for three years before she took another job in Baltimore Broadcasting Station –where there were larger market segment and greater prestige and challenge as well. This step later proved to be the biggest blessing in disguise mistake Oprah had made.

Oprah was usually calm and self-controlled in her previous job, but now she looked so exhausted. She forgot to read the text copy prior to her appearance before the camera. She misspelled "blasé" and misplaced Barbados to be somewhere in California and made a small laugh at that incident. She interviewed a fire victim with such style as asking "How did you feel after the ordeal?" then wept in front of the camera and apologized for exploiting woman's emotion. The station management did not appreciate her attitude in front of the camera and they didn't like her appearance either. They complained about her hair style, her big nose and the distance between her eyes. Tempted to glamorize her appearance, they sent her to a good salon in New York which did a disastrous remodeling that made her hair fall off. Failing to find a suitable wig, she managed to appear on the camera (then she said: "You will learn a lot about yourself if you are baldheaded, a black and a news broadcaster in Baltimore")
In one year her glory was to be unpredictably coming.

The station had had enough of this new figure. They decided she just didn't fit to TV news broadcasting job. But to avoid breaking her contract, they choose not to fire her but lowered her position from broadcaster to presenter of a talk show for housewives called "People Are Talking" run at daytime. Oprah said, "Failure is the way God chooses to remind you that you are on the wrong track". But clearly she is now on the right track about her first day on the talk show "it is like a breath of relief, and it is exactly what you must feel". The show was a prime show and most of the audience were women who found themselves reflected in the figure of that simple, direct, funny and human presenter. Seven years later, Oprah's show attracted a station in Chicago and she was offered to move there to direct the A. M. Chicago show.

In a month, she made that show the most loveable show. In 1985 the show was further developed and given a new name: The Oprah Winfrey Show and is now nationally broadcasted. During more than 15 years of unpredicted success, Oprah keep sharing many things, including her own struggle and success affairs:

going on a diet against too much food and fat (she eventually got her ideal weight), a law suit by a ranch owner (which she won), the "TV Garbage" program which dominates her market segment (she soared up and achieved highest rating). Even after all she had been through, she refused to see her failures as mistakes. "I don't believe in failure" Oprah said. "It is not a failure if you enjoy the process".

Once upon a time, a farmer owned an old mule who tripped and fell into the farmer's well. The farmer heard the mule braying and was unable to figure out how to bring up the old animal. It grieved him that he could not pull the animal out. He'd been a good worker around the farm. Although the farmer sympathized with the mule, he called his neighbors together and told them what had happened. He had them help haul dirt to bury the old mule in the well and quietly put him out of his misery.
At first, the old mule was puzzled, but as the farmer and his neighbors continued shoveling and the dirt hit his back, he had a thought: he ought to shake off the dirt and step up. And he did just that.

"Shake it off and step up...shake it off and step up...shake it off and step up." Even though he took painful blows of dirt and fought panic, he just kept right on shaking it off and stepping up! It wasn't long before the old mule stepped up and over the lip of that well. What could have buried him actually blessed him...all because of the manner in which he handled his adversity.

Once upon a time, a daughter complained to her father that her life was miserable and that she didn't know how she was going to make it. She was tired of fighting and struggling all the time. It seemed just as one problem was solved, another one soon followed. Her father, a chef, took her to the kitchen. He filled three pots with water and placed each on a high fire. Once the three pots began to boil, he placed potatoes in one pot, eggs in the second pot, and ground coffee beans in the third pot. He then let them sit and boil, without saying a word to his daughter. The daughter moaned and impatiently waited, wondering what he was doing. After twenty minutes, he turned off the burners. He took the potatoes out of the pot and placed them in a bowl. He pulled the eggs out and placed them in a bowl. He then ladled the coffee out and placed it in a cup. Turning to her, he asked, "Daughter, what do you see?" "Potatoes, eggs, and coffee," she hastily replied. "Look closer", he said, "and touched the potatoes". She did and noted that they were soft. He then asked her to take an egg and break it. After pulling off the shell, she observed the hard-boiled egg. Finally, he asked her to sip the coffee. Its rich aroma brought a smile
to her face. "Father, what does this mean?" she asked.
He then explained that the potatoes, the eggs, and coffee beans had each faced the same adversity, the boiling water. However, each one reacted differently.
The potato went in strong, hard and unrelenting, but in boiling water it became soft and weak. The egg was fragile

with the thin outer shell protecting its liquid interior until it was put in the boiling water. Then the inside of the egg became hard. However, the ground coffee beans were unique. After they were exposed to the boiling water, they changed the water and created something new. "Which are you?" he asked his daughter. "When adversity knocks on your door, how do you respond? Are you a potato, an egg, or a coffee bean?" In life, things happen around us and things happen to us, but the only thing that truly matters is what happens within us.

When things go wrong as they sometimes will
When the road you're trudging seems all up hill.
When funds are low and the debts are high.
And you want to smile, but you have to sigh.
When care is pressing you down a bit.
Rest, if you must, but don't you quit.
Life is queer with its twists and turns.
As every one of us sometimes learns.
And many a failure turns about
When he might have won had he stuck it out.
Don't give up though the pace seems slow -
You may succeed with another blow.
Success is failure turned inside out -
The silver tint of the clouds of doubt.
And you never can tell how close you are.
It may be near when it seems so far:
So stick to the fight when you're hardest hit
It's when things seem worst that you must not quit.

People are unreasonable, illogical, and self-centered.

LOVE THEM ANYWAY.

If you do good, people accuse you of selfish, ulterior motives.

DO GOOD ANYWAY.

If you are successful, you win false and true enemies.

SUCCEED ANYWAY.

The good you do will be forgotten tomorrow.

DO GOOD ANYWAY.

Honesty and frankness make you vulnerable.

BE HONEST AND FRANK ANYWAY.

What you spent years building may be destroyed overnight.

BUILD ANYWAY.

People really need help but may attack you if you help them.

HELP PEOPLE ANYWAY.

Give the world the best you have and you'll get kicked in the teeth.

GIVE THE WORLD THE BEST YOU'VE GOT ANYWAY.

An elderly couple retired to the countryside to a small isolated cottage overlooking some rugged and rocky heathland. One early morning, the woman saw from her window a young man dressed in working clothes walking on the heath about a hundred yards away. He was carrying a spade and a small case and he disappeared from view behind a copse of trees. The woman thought no more about it but around the same time the next day she saw the man again, carrying his spade and a small case, and again he disappeared behind the copse. The woman mentioned this to her husband who said he was probably a farmer or gamekeeper setting traps, or performing some other country practice that would be perfectly normal, and so not to worry. However, after several more sightings of the young man with the spade over the next two weeks, the woman persuaded her husband to take a stroll - early, before the man tended to arrive - to the copse of trees to investigate what he was doing. There they found a surprisingly long and deep trench, rough and uneven at one end, becoming much neater and tidier towards the other end.

"How strange," the old lady said, "Why dig a trench here...and in such difficult rocky ground?" and her husband agreed. Just then the young man appeared earlier than his usual time.

"You're early," said the old woman, making light of their obvious curiosity, "We wondered what you were doing and we also wondered what was in the case." "I'm digging a trench," said the man who continued, realizing a bigger explanation was appropriate. "I'm actually learning how to dig a good trench because the job I'm being interviewed for later today says that experience is essential, so I'm getting the experience. And the case...it's got my lunch in it."
He got the job.

DETERMINATON

In 1883, a creative engineer named John Roebling was inspired by an idea to build a spectacular bridge connecting New York with the Long Island. However bridge building experts throughout the world thought that this was an impossible feat and told Roebling to forget the idea. It just could not be done. It was not practical. It had never been done before. Roebling could not ignore the vision he had in his mind of this bridge. He thought about it all the time and he knew deep in his heart that it could be done. He just had to share the dream with someone else. After much discussion and persuasion he managed to convince his son Washington, an up and coming engineer, that the bridge in fact could be built. Working together for the first time, the father and son developed concepts of how it could be accomplished and how the obstacles could be overcome. With great excitement and inspiration, and the headiness of a wild challenge before them, they hired their crew and began to build their dream bridge.

The project started well, but when it was only a few months underway a tragic accident on the site took the life of John Roebling. Washington was injured and left with a certain amount of brain damage, which resulted in him not being able to walk or talk or even move. "We told them so." "Crazy men and their crazy dreams." "It`s foolish to chase wild visions."

Everyone had a negative comment to make and felt that the project should be scrapped since the Roebling's were the only ones who knew how the bridge could be built. In spite of his handicap Washington was never discouraged and still had a burning desire to complete the bridge and his mind was still as sharp as ever. He tried to inspire and pass on his enthusiasm to some of his friends, but they were too daunted by the task. As he lay on his bed in his hospital room, with the sunlight streaming through the windows, a gentle breeze blew the flimsy white curtains apart and he was able to see the sky and the tops of the trees outside for just a moment. It seemed that there was a message for him not to give up. Suddenly an idea hit him. All he could do was move one finger and he decided to make the best use of it. By moving this, he slowly developed a code of communication with his wife.

He touched his wife's arm with that finger, indicating to her that he wanted her to call the engineers again. Then he used the same method of tapping her arm to tell the engineers what to do. It seemed foolish but the project was under way again. For 13 years Washington tapped out his instructions with his finger on his wife's arm, until the bridge was finally completed. Today the spectacular Brooklyn Bridge stands in all its glory as a tribute to the triumph of one man's indomitable spirit and his determination not to be defeated by circumstances. It is also a tribute to the engineers and their team work, and to their faith in a man who was considered mad by half the world. It stands too as a tangible monument to the love and devotion of his wife who for 13 long years patiently decoded the messages of her husband and told the engineers what to do.

Perhaps this is one of the best examples of a never-say-die attitude that overcomes a terrible physical handicap and achieves an impossible goal. Often when we face obstacles in our day-to-day life, our hurdles seem very small in comparison to what many others have to face. The Brooklyn Bridge shows us that dreams that seem impossible can be realized with determination and persistence, no matter what the odds are. Even the most distant dream can be realized with determination and persistence.

Chapter 3: Generosity

Mahatma Gandhi went from city to city, village to village collecting funds for the Charkha Sangh. During one of his tours he addressed a meeting in Orissa. After his speech a poor old woman got up. She was bent with age, her hair was grey and her clothes were in tatters. The volunteers tried to stop her, but she fought her way to the place where Gandhiji was sitting. "I must see him," she insisted and going up to Gandhiji touched his feet. Then from the folds of her sari she brought out a copper coin and placed it at his feet. Gandhiji picked up the copper coin and put it away carefully. The Charkha Sangh funds were under the charge of Jamnalal Bajaj. He asked Gandhiji for the coin but Gandhiji refused. "I keep cheques worth thousands of rupees for the Charkha Sangh," Jamnalal Bajaj said laughingly "yet you won't trust me with a copper coin." "This copper coin is worth much more than those thousands," Gandhiji said. "If a man has several lakhs and he gives away a thousand or two, it doesn't mean much. But this coin was perhaps all that the poor woman possessed. She gave me all she had. That was very generous of her. What a great sacrifice she made. That is why I value this copper coin more than a crore of rupees." To rejoice about.

The Window

Two men, both seriously ill, occupied the same hospital room. One man was allowed to sit up in his bed for an hour a day to drain the fluids from his lungs. His bed was next to the room's only window. The other man had to spend all his time flat on his back. The men talked for hours on end. They spoke of their wives and families, their homes, their jobs, their involvement in the military service, where they had been on vacation. And every afternoon when the man in the bed next to the window could sit up, he would pass the time by describing to his roommate all the things he could see outside the window.

The man in the other bed would live for those one-hour periods where his world would be broadened and enlivened by all the activity and color of the outside world. The window overlooked a park with a lovely lake, the man had said. Ducks and swans played on the water while children sailed their model boats. Lovers walked arm in arm amid flowers of every color of the rainbow. Grand old trees graced the landscape, and a fine view of the city skyline could be seen in the distance. As the man by the window described all this in exquisite detail, the man on the other side of the room would close his eyes and imagine the picturesque scene.

One warm afternoon the man by the window described a parade passing by. Although the other man could not hear the band, he could see it in his mind's eye as the gentleman by the window portrayed it with descriptive words. Unexpectedly, an alien thought entered his head: Why should he have all the pleasure of seeing everything while I never get to see anything? It didn't seem fair. As the thought fermented, the man felt ashamed at first. But as the days passed and he missed seeing more sights, his envy eroded into resentment and soon turned him sour. He began to brood and found himself unable to sleep. He should be by that window - and that thought now controlled his life.

Late one night, as he lay staring at the ceiling, the man by the window began to cough. He was choking on the fluid in his lungs. The other man watched in the dimly lit room as the struggling man by the window groped for the button to call for help. Listening from across the room, he never moved, never pushed his own button, which would have brought the nurse running. In less than five minutes, the coughing and choking stopped, along with the sound of breathing.

Now, there was only silence--deathly silence.
The following morning, the day nurse arrived to bring water for their baths. When she found the lifeless body of the man by the window, she was saddened and called the hospital attendant to take it away--no words, no fuss. As soon as it seemed appropriate, the man asked if
he could be moved next to the window. The nurse was happy to make the switch and after making sure he was comfortable, she left him alone. Slowly, painfully, he propped himself up on one elbow to take his first look. Finally, he would have the joy of seeing it all himself. He strained to slowly turn to look out the window beside the bed. It faced a blank wall.

Moral of the story:

The pursuit of happiness is a matter of choice...it is a positive attitude we consciously choose to express. It is not a gift that gets delivered to our doorstep each morning, nor does it come through the window. And I am certain that our circumstances are just a small part of what makes us joyful. If we wait for them to get just right, we will never find lasting joy. The pursuit of happiness is an inward journey. Our minds are like programs, awaiting the code that will determine behaviors; like bank vaults awaiting our deposits. If we regularly deposit positive, encouraging, and uplifting thoughts, if we continue to bite our lips just before we begin to grumble and complain, if we shoot down that seemingly harmless negative thought as it germinates, we will find that there is much.

The Starfish

There was a man taking a morning walk at or the beach. He saw that along with the morning tide came hundreds of starfish and when they would die. The tide was fresh and the starfish were alive. The man took a few steps, picked one and threw it into the water. He did that repeatedly. Right behind him there was another person who couldn't understand what this man was doing. He caught up with him and asked, "What are you doing? There are hundreds of starfish. How many can you help? What difference does it make?" This man did not reply, took two more steps, picked up another one, threw it into the water, and said, "It makes a difference to this one."

Unconditional Love

A motivating story a story is told about a soldier who was finally coming home after having fought in Vietnam. He called his parents from San Francisco. "Mom and Dad, I'm coming home, but I've a favor to ask. I have a friend I'd like to bring home with me." "Sure," they replied, "we'd love to meet him." "There's something you should know the son continued, "he was hurt pretty badly in the fighting. He stepped on a land mind and lost an arm and a leg. He has nowhere else to go, and I want him to come live with us." Friends are a very rare jewel, indeed. They make you smile and encourage you to succeed they lend an ear, they share a word of praise, and they always want to open their hearts to us.

Don't We All?

I was parked in front of the mall wiping off my car. I had just come from the car wash and was waiting for my wife to get out of work. Coming my way from across the parking lot was what society would consider a bum. From the looks of him, he had no car, no home, no clean clothes, and no money. There are times when you feel generous but there are other times that you just don't want to be bothered. This was one of those "don't want to be bothered times." "I hope he doesn't ask me for any money," I thought. He didn't. He came and sat on the curb in front of the bus stop but he didn't look like he could have enough money to even ride the bus. After a few minutes he spoke. "That's a very pretty car," he said. He was ragged but he had an air of dignity around him. His scraggly blond beard keep more than his face warm. I said, "thanks," and continued wiping off my car. He sat there quietly as I worked. The expected plea for money never came. As the silence between us widened something inside said, "ask him if he needs any help." I was sure that he would say "yes" but I held true to the inner voice. "Do you need any help?" I asked. He answered in three simple but profound words that I shall never forget.

We often look for wisdom in great men and women. We expect it from those of higher learning and accomplishments. I expected nothing but an outstretched grimy hand. He spoke the three words that shook me. "Don't we all?" he said. I was feeling high and mighty, successful and important, above a bum in the street, until those three words hit me like a twelve gauge shotgun. Don't we all? I needed help. Maybe not for bus fare or a place to sleep, but I needed help. I reached in my wallet and gave him not only enough for bus fare, but enough to get a warm meal and shelter for the day. Those three little words still ring true. No matter how much you have, no matter how much you have accomplished, you need help too. No matter how little you have, no matter how loaded you are with problems, even without money or a place to sleep, you can give help. Even if it's just a compliment, you can give that. You never know when you may see someone that appears to have it all. They are waiting on you to give them what they don't have. A different perspective on life, a glimpse at something beautiful, a respite from daily chaos, which only you through a torn world can see. Maybe the man was just a homeless stranger wandering the streets. Maybe he was more than that.

Maybe he was sent by a power that is great and wise, to minister to a soul too comfortable in themselves. Maybe God looked down, called an Angel, dressed him like a bum, then said, "go minister to that man cleaning the car, that man needs help." Don't we all?

How would you like to be remembered?

About a hundred years ago, a man looked at the morning newspaper and to his surprise and horror, read his name in the obituary column. The newspapers had reported the death of the wrong person by mistake. His first response was shock. Am I here or there? When he regained his composure, his second thought was to find out what people had said about him. The obituary read, "Dynamite King Dies." And also "He was the merchant of death." This man was the inventor of dynamite and when he read the words "merchant of death," he asked himself a question, "Is this how I am going to be remembered?" He got in touch with his feelings and decided that this was not the way he wanted to be remembered. From that day on, he started working toward peace. His name was Alfred Nobel and he is remembered today by the great Nobel Prize. Just as Alfred Nobel got in touch with his feelings and redefined his values, we should step back and do the same.

What is your legacy?

How would you like to be remembered?
Will you be spoken well of?
Will you be remembered with love and respect?
Will you be missed?

The Midas Touch

We all know the story of the greedy king named Midas. He had a lot of gold and the more he had the more he wanted. He stored all the gold in his vaults and used to spend time every day counting it. One day while he was counting a stranger came from nowhere and said he would grant him a wish. The king was delighted and said, "I would like everything I touch to turn to gold." The stranger asked the king, Are you sure?" The king replied, "Yes." So the stranger said, "Starting tomorrow morning with the sun rays you will get the golden touch." The king thought he must be dreaming, this couldn't be true. But the next day when he woke up, he touched the bed, his clothes, and everything turned to gold. He looked out of the window and saw his daughter playing in the garden. He decided to give her a surprise and thought she would be happy. But before he went to the garden he decided to read a book.

The moment he touched it, it turned into gold and he couldn't read it. Then he sat to have breakfast and the moment he touched the fruit and the glass of water, they turned to gold. He was getting hungry and he said to himself, "I can't eat and drink gold". Just about that time his daughter came running and he hugged her and she turned into a gold statue. There were no more smiles left. The king bowed his head and started crying. The stranger who gave the wish came again and asked the king if he was happy with his golden touch. The king said he was the most miserable man. The stranger asked, "What would you rather have, your food and loving daughter or lumps of gold and her golden statue?" The king cried and asked for forgiveness. He said, "I will give up all my gold. Please give me my daughter back because without her I have lost everything worth having." The stranger said to the king, "You have become wiser than before" and he reversed the spell. He got his daughter back.

Meaningless Goals

A farmer had a dog who used to sit by the roadside waiting for vehicles to come around. As soon as one came he would run down the road, barking and trying to overtake it. One day a neighbor asked the farmer "Do you think your dog is ever going to catch a car?" The farmer replied, "That is not what bothers me. What bothers me is what he would do if he ever caught one." Many people in life behave like that dog who is pursuing meaningless goals. In his arms and the king learned a lesson that he never forget for the rest of his life.

Which Road

A man was traveling and stopped at an intersection. He asked an elderly man, "Where does this road take me?" The elderly person asked, "Where do you want to go?" The man replied, "I don't know." The elderly person said, "Then take any road. What difference does it make?"

Chapter 4: Inspirational Women Stories

Inspirational Women Stories From Around The World

The what? The Strongwoman competition? Kara Mann wasn't what I expected. Nor did I expect to be so fascinated and so inspired by a 23-year-old. Her look, demeanor and voice were not unlike one of the cheerleaders she has had to dead-lift in competition. Another stereotype bites the dust.

In 2004, Kara Mann became the National Strongwoman Champion, less than two years after first starting to compete in the sport. After winning that competition again as recently as 2006, she is now a two time national champ. Where did she come from and how did she get there so fast? A native of Boston, she first got into it through a boyfriend and his family who encouraged her to give it a try. Her ascent was rapid, beginning with third place in the Massachusetts state championships. Mann shook her head when asked if she would have done anything differently, having been a three-sport athlete in high school where she succeeded at cross-country, basketball and track and field, and dabbled in gymnastics, taekwondo and playing the flute.

Today she uses her degree from Vanderbilt in chemical engineering at her job at General Electric in Cleveland and is learning to juggle her vocation and her strongwoman hobby. "You can't do it as a career." When asked about financial rewards, she laughed. "Sometimes they give us swords, Samurai swords. Once I did get three hundred dollars, though."

So why would someone so physically strong, athletic and focused choose this? The well-known health benefits of this level of physical conditioning aside, "It's a passion. It's a release of energy and stress for me…and you can't imagine the highs, the empowering feeling you get after being successful in a competition." Asked to describe a typical competition, her eyes light up. "You never know what to expect." The unpredictable nature of each competition holds particular appeal for Mann. What is consistent about the competitions is that three aspects of skill and strength are always tested: "overhead," "grip" (e.g., see how long you can keep two Mini Cooper cars from rolling) and "back and legs."

In addition, one can always expect the classic, signature event called Atlas Stones, where contestants carry large cement stones of varying weight and shape over to a platform. She once pulled an A-4 military airplane 47 feet in 60 seconds. A typical week involves strength training each weekday, followed by "implement" training on the weekends. Implement training zeroes in on the specific mechanical skills involved in the upcoming events. In the week preceding an event, the amount of implement training increases. In all three geographic settings of her life, Boston, Nashville and now Cleveland, she has connected to a network of athletes with this pursuit, most of them males, who she refers to as if they were her brothers. Just as important as physical preparation is mental preparation. She is convinced that the quality of her mental focus at the time of her event is crucial. "You can't be distracted in the least or paying attention to your opponents." Mann uses what she calls "angry" music, like Disturbed, to get her psyched and ready. "I don't even know what they're saying." She attributes her success in putting mind over matter to her upbringing and to her experience in other sports.

Behind this modest, casual, relaxed demeanor, there lies a woman with strong opinions about what is wrong with the sport. She laments that there are but a handful of females who compete consistently. The corollary to that problem is the lack of financial rewards. She would like to see the women break off from the male federation, recognizing a need for more woman-power in the decision-making. She would like more consistency, predictability and regularity in dates and locations of competitions. And perhaps most importantly, she would like to see the sport regulated. Right now there is no drug-testing whatsoever in either the male or female milieus. "I really have issues with that, since it constitutes an uneven playing field." Mann's goal is to attract other females to this sport that she loves, and along with that, to inspire entrants to compete without "supplements." She even envisions two separate classes for those who "do" and those who "don't." All of these improvements would help to shift strongwoman away from its entertainment flavor toward its status as a serious "sport."

You can bet that Kara Mann, at 5'6" and 165 pounds, will be a force in helping shape the evolution of her sport. She's just that strong.

Eileen Marie Collins (Colonel, USAF, RET.) NASA Astronaut

Born November 19, 1956, in Elmira , New York.
Eileen graduated from Elmira Free Academy, Elmira, New York, in 1974 and received an Associate in Science degree in mathematics/science from Corning Community College in 1976. She went on to earn a Bachelor of Arts degree in mathematics and economics from Syracuse University in 1978. She also has a Master of Science degree in operations research from Stanford University in

1986 and a Master of Arts degree in space systems management from Webster University in 1989. As a small girl she gazed up into the sky and watched the silent birds (sailplanes) soar through the air, this is where the love affair began. Eileen grew up in the "Soaring Capital of America." She was fascinated with flight and knew that one day she wanted to fly. At the age of 19 she had saved $1,000 and went to her local airport to ask them to show her how to fly. Her inspiration was fueled by women pilots and early astronauts. Through years of education, determination and hard work she has logged more than 6,751 hours in both the air and space! Eileen joined the Air Force and began pilot training in 1978, the same year that NASA opened the Shuttle program to women. She became an official astronaut in 1991.

Eileen Collins is the first and currently only female Space Shuttle Commander in history!! Four space flights and 872 hours in space later Eileen retired from NASA in May 2006.

Battling dyslexia

Rebecca, who I met at a business conference in Las Vegas, is one of the smartest people I know. Even if you were around her for an entire day, you probably wouldn't notice her disability. "I was born with severe dyslexia," Rebecca explains. "Due to my learning disability, I was in special education classes for most of my elementary and middle school years." Despite the challenge, she refused to let dyslexia dictate her life. Every day, she worked on overcoming her disability with the help of her parents. "My dad would spend an hour every morning helping me with math," says Rebecca. "In the evenings, my mom would have me read books out loud and then she would quiz me on the content." Rebecca's hard work paid off. By high school, she had advanced from special education classes all the way to honors classes. When high school came to an end, she kept striving. "When I was a young, no one thought I could ever go to college," she confides. Not only did Rebecca end up going to college, she graduated near the top of her class. Was her journey over? Hardly. "I always had a vision," says Rebecca, "of one day being a lawyer. But it seemed like such a crazy aspiration that I never told anyone."

Today, Rebecca's vision is a reality. She graduated from law school and is currently working her way up in one of the largest law firms on the East Coast. Rebecca says: "I wouldn't change a thing. My learning disability still makes life a challenge but it also gave me the determination to make my dream come true."

"Mom, why are you crying?" he asked his mom. "Because I'm a woman" she told him. "I don't understand," he said. His mom just hugged him and said, "and you never will." Later the little boy asked his father, "Why does mother seem to cry for no reason?" "All women cry for no reason" was all his dad could say. The little boy grew up and became a man, still wondering why women cry. Finally he put in a call to GOD. When GOD got on the phone the man said, "GOD, why do women cry so easily?" GOD said: "When I made women she had to be special. I made her shoulders strong enough to carry the weight of the world; yet, gentle enough to give comfort. I gave her an inner strength to endure childbirth and the rejection that many times comes from her children. I gave her a hardness that allows her to keep going when everyone else gives up and take care of her family through sickness and fatigue without complaining. I gave her the sensitivity to love her children under any and all circumstances, even when her child has hurt her very badly. This same sensitivity helps her to make a child's boo-boo feel better and shares in her teenager's anxieties and fears. I gave her strength to carry her husband through his faults and fashioned her from his rib to protect his heart. I gave her wisdom to know that a good husband never hurts his wife, but sometimes tests her strengths and her resolve to stand beside him unfalteringly. I gave her a tear to shed, it's hers exclusively to use whenever it is needed. It's her only weakness; it's a tear for mankind."

Yasmin Waljee, 38, a lawyer, from London

Yasmin will never meet all the thousands of people she has helped. But her belief that justice is a right for all - and that the disadvantaged who can't access a diminishing legal aid system should be represented for free by some of Britain's top lawyers - drives her relentlessly on. Yasmin, is head of Pro Bono - provision of free service by volunteer lawyers - at top legal firm Lovells. She helps mastermind 18,000 free hours of legal help a year worldwide - from victims of domestic violence, victims of terrorist attacks including the London July 7 bombings, disabled people who are fighting for Disability Living Allowance and desperate families facing eviction in East London because they are falling behind with rent.

While Yasmin - married with a one-year-old son - claims modestly that all the above is not her work alone, she also tirelessly raises money for charity: for example, persuading her colleagues to abseil down their building and arranging a team of lawyers to help clean up a rundown area of Newham, East London. Last year, working with a committee of staff, she raised £25,000 for Save The Children through Legally Ballroom Dancing - an event which saw 30 lawyers waltzing in front of their colleagues.

Chapter 5: Teachings from Animals

Teachings and Lessons from Animals

A lady takes her pet Chihuahua with her on a safari holiday. Wandering too far one day the Chihuahua gets lost in the bush, and soon encounters a very hungry looking leopard. The Chihuahua realizes he's in trouble, but, noticing some fresh bones on the ground, he settles down to chew on them, with his back to the big cat. As the leopard is about to leap, the Chihuahua smacks his lips and exclaims loudly, "Boy, that was one delicious leopard. I wonder if there are any more around here." The leopard stops mid-stride, and slinks away into the trees. "Phew," says the leopard", that was close - that evil little dog nearly had me". A monkey nearby sees everything and thinks he'll win a favor by putting the stupid leopard straight. The Chihuahua sees the monkey go after the leopard, and guesses he might be up to no good. When the leopard hears the monkey's story he feels angry at being made a fool, and offers the monkey a ride back to see him exact his revenge. The little dog sees them approaching and fears the worse. Thinking quickly, the little dog turns his back, pretends not to notice them, and when the pair are within earshot says aloud, "Now where's that monkey got to? I sent him ages ago to bring me another leopard..."

Two frogs fell into a deep pit, and though they tried very hard they could not hop out. Their comrades peered down from the top and croaked in sympathy. "We feel for you," they shouted, "but there's no way you can get out from there!" On hearing this, one of the frogs lost heart, and died of fear. The other frog was deaf. He thought his comrades were shouting encouragement. Emboldened by their faith in him, he gathered up all his reserves of energy in one great jump that landed him out of the pit.

Hang on to your own bone

Fanny the farm dog was pretty smart, but one day she got the shock of her life because no-one had ever told her about mirrors. As a special treat, she was given a big bone. She took it down to the river bank to enjoy it in peace. As she stood there with the bone in her mouth, she looked at her reflection in the water. And what did she see? Another dog with a bone in its mouth! She wanted the other bone as well as her own, so she opened her mouth to bark and her bone fell straight in and sank to the bottom.

The rooster makes its last mistake

Two burglars were prowling round a barn one night. They could hear something moving inside, and ever so carefully they climbed in to see what it was. It was a rooster. "Ah-ha," they cried. "This will do for our supper tomorrow." They grabbed it and were about to kill it when the rooster squawked in alarm: "Please don't kill me. I can be useful to you. I can wake you at dawn every day, ready to start work on time." "That's just what we don't want," growled the burglars. "If you wake people up they'll catch us robbing their houses." So that was the end of the rooster.

The jealous goat

A goat and a donkey lived on the same farm. The goat had to find his own food, but because he made the donkey work hard, the farmer fed him. The goat became jealous, forgetting all the donkey's hard work. He thought if the donkey stopped working, he would get his food. So he pushed him into a large hole, and he was badly hurt. The farmer sent for the vet, who examined the donkey. "The quickest way to make him better," he said, "is to feed him with goat soup." So instead of getting the donkey's food for himself, the goat finished up as food for the donkey!

Look before you eat

You know what dogs are like. If you drop a bit of food from the table they shallow it before they know what it is. But sometimes they wish they hadn't. Fanny the farm dog wasn't allowed in while her master Josh was eating with the family. But one day she crept in and hid under the table when no-one was looking. She kept very quiet until suddenly a big dollop of food fell next to her. She gobbled it up without thinking. Then she let out a big howl and rushed outside, holding her tummy with one paw. The family was eating a very hot curry for supper!

One good turn deserves another

Fred was a farm-worker who found a young eagle caught in a trap. He couldn't bear to see such a beautiful bird in pain, so he released it. A few days later, he was sitting in the shade of an old wall, having bread and cheese for his lunch. Suddenly, with a flapping of wings, the eagle swooped and stole the cap from his head. It flew away just above the ground with Fred rushing after it, shouting, until it dropped his cap. Fred put it back on his head and trudged back to finish his lunch. But what do you think? Exactly where he had been sitting the old wall had collapsed! Each of them had saved the other.

How to live in peace

In the old days, farmers sometimes encouraged snakes and weasels to live in the barn and kill the mice that ate their corn. But on one farm there was a bad-tempered weasel and a peppery old snake, and instead of killing the mice they kept fighting each other. The mice thought this was wonderful, of course. At first, they just put their heads cautiously out of their holes to watch. Before long, they began to form a circle around the two fighters and cheer for one side or the other. For a while, the snake and the weasel were so busy scrapping they didn't even notice. One day, however, they stopped for a rest in the middle of a particularly tiring fight. They looked around them and then at each other. "Why are we wasting so much eating time," they asked themselves. "There's enough food here to make us fat and good-tempered." And they set about gobbling up the mice.

Animals Are Parents Too

I want to let you know about an event that changed my life many years ago. It is a memory that periodically comes and goes, but it is one of the most precious memories that me and my wife share. I am thankful that we can remember it together. It's a reminder that things are not what they seem and that angels come in many packages. We live in College Station, Texas and we were on our way home from Houston, Texas around the Weston Lakes area one Saturday or Sunday morning. And when I say morning, I'm talking 1:00 to 2:00 in the morning. We were on our way home and decided to stop at a local gas station to get coffee and something to snack on since it was a good hour and a half before we got home. When we were done, we got back into our car and before I started it, we noticed a man standing outside in front of the building. You could tell that he was a homeless man. His clothes were tattered and worn and it looked like he had gone in and gotten him some coffee or something warm to drink since it was cold this time of the year. He must have not had enough money to get something to eat. That is not something I remember too well, because that is not what "moved" me. The next thing I remember is a dog that walked up to the front of the building. Being a dog lover, I noticed that she was part wolf and probably part German shepherd. I could tell she was a she, because you could tell that she had been feeding puppies. She was terribly in need of something to eat and I felt so bad for her. I knew if she didn't eat soon, she and her puppies would not make it.

Me and my wife sat there and looked at her. We noticed that people walked by and didn't even pet her, like most people do when they walk by an animal in front of a store. She might not have been as pretty and clean as most, but she still deserved better. But we still did not do anything. But someone did. The homeless man, who I thought did not buy himself anything to eat, went back into the store. And what he did brought tears to me and my wife. He had gone into the store and with what money he may have had, bought a can of dog food and fed that dog. I know that this story isn't as inspirational as most stories, but it plays a great part in our lives. You see, that was Mother's Day weekend. And a lot of people forget that some animals are parents too. And animals as well as us are God's creations too. It would be a better story if I could remember all the details, but even without the details, I believe it still gets the message across. It took a homeless man, to show me what I should have done. He made me a better man that day.

Sweltering temperatures are a reminder to keep not only yourselves cool, but your pets. In the case of a Labrador, he may have been left alone, but helped himself survive what could have been a terrible situation. Eleven-year-old Max is not just a dog. He's like another member of Donna Gardner's family. "You have to know Max. He's a very smart dog and he just does things that I don't think a normal dog does all the time," said Gardner. The chocolate Lab proved that a couple of weeks ago. Gardner ran an errand and took Max with her. When she came home a short time later, she went inside the house, forgetting Max was still in the car. "I came in and started cleaning and about an hour later I heard a horn blow," said Gardner. She went outside, but didn't see anybody. "So I came back in the house and I started cleaning again and the horn blew again." This time, she saw Max sitting in her driver's seat. "I rushed over and got him out real fast and he was panting like crazy. I brought him in the house and he just dropped to the floor," Gardner said. Gardner gave him water and cooled him down. Her daughter called the vet who said Max was a little weak, a little slow but otherwise OK.

"Number 1... Max saved his own life by honking the horn to get himself out of a very, very overheated car. Number 2, the Gardners are such good pet owners that they looked at him first. They managed to get his temperature down a little bit before they got here," said Nancy Soares with the Macungie Animal Hospital. "I don't know whatever made me forget he was with me," added Gardner. Meanwhile, Gardner says she will never make that mistake again and hopes this serves as a lesson to other pet parents.

Bernadetta Henry suffers from sleep apnea, which affects her airways and causes her to stop breathing several times each night. Bernadetta Henry and Boris, who acts as a hearing dog. Faithful Boris lies next to the grandmother as she sleeps and carefully monitors her life-threatening condition through the night. The bichon frise listens out for her - and puts his paw on her chest to wake her when her breathing stops. 'He means everything to me. If it wasn't for him, I would be dead,' said Mrs Henry, from Llangollen,

Denbighshire, in north-east Wales. Boris has been her hearing dog since she became almost completely deaf as a result of a blood clot. Mrs Henry later had an allergic reaction to the blood-thinning drug warfarin, resulting in a brain hemorrhage. After physiotherapy, she was confined to a wheelchair, making her more dependent on her family. But, since the death of her husband five years ago, Mrs Henry, who is in her 70s, has been reliant on Boris and depends on him to alert her when the phone or doorbell rings and when the cooker's timer goes off.

'I couldn't live on my own without him and we both love each other. He's full of fun and can be very mischievous,' she said.

A 68-year-old violin maker from Zagreb has been saved from certain death after his dog alerted neighbors when he fell into an insulin comma. Krsto Pekic was saved after his dog Rex began banging on the front door and making enough noise for neighbors to hear him. They called police and fire fighters who broke into the apartment and took the unconscious Pekic to hospital. He is currently recovering in Sestre Milosrdnice Hospital in Zagreb and is out of danger, the Croatian daily Vecernji List reports.

Wrapping Up

Wow! Do you feel inspired? That was a great run-through a huge collection of inspiring stories from around the world! We all have our own stories. It is up to us, whether we want to live extraordinary lives which inspire and motivate each other or not. Even animals, in the last chapter have showed us that their courage is worth modeling. Let us strive to give our fullest gifts to the world and make the world a better place! It is with great hope that this collection of stories has inspired you and encouraged you to spread the love to your readers. To your success!

Poems That Inspire

If-Rudyard Kipling

If you can keep your head when all about you
Are losing theirs and blaming it on you.
If you can trust yourself when all men doubt you,
But make allowance for their doubting too;
If you can wait and not be tired by waiting,
Or being lied about, don't deal in lies,
Or being hated, don't give way to hating,
And yet don't look too good, nor talk too wise:
If you can dream - and not make dreams your master;
If you can think - and not make thoughts your aim;
If you can meet with Triumph and Disaster
And treat these two impostors just the same;
If you can bear to hear the truth you've spoken
Twisted by knaves to make a trap for fools,
Or watch the things you gave your life to, broken,
And stoop and build 'em up with worn-out tools:
If you can make one heap of all your winnings
And risk it on one turn of pitch-and-toss,
And lose, and start again at your beginnings
And never breathe a word about your loss;
If you can force your heart and nerve and sinew
To serve your turn long after they are gone,
And so hold on when there is nothing in you
Except the Will which says to them: 'Hold on!'
If you can talk with crowds and keep your virtue,
Or walk with Kings - nor lose the common touch,
If neither foes nor loving friends can hurt you,
If all men count with you, but none too much;
If you can fill the unforgiving minute
With sixty seconds' worth of distance run,
Yours is the Earth and everything that's in it,

And - which is more - you'll be a Man, my son!

The Road Not Taken-Robert Frost

Two roads diverged in a yellow wood,
And sorry I could not travel both
And be one traveler, long I stood
And looked down one as far as I could
To where it bent in the undergrowth.
Then took the other, as just as fair,
And having perhaps the better claim,
Because it was grassy and wanted wear;
Though as for that the passing there
Had worn them really about the same.
And both that morning equally lay
In leaves no step had trodden black.
Oh, I kept the first for another day!
Yet knowing how way leads on to way,
I doubted if I should ever come back.
I shall be telling this with a sigh
Somewhere ages and ages hence:
Two roads diverged in a wood, and I--
I took the one less travelled by,
And that has made all the difference.

It Couldn't be Done-Edgar Guest

Somebody said that it couldn't be done,
But, he with a chuckle replied
That "maybe it couldn't" but he would be one
Who wouldn't say so till he'd tried?
So he buckled right in with the trace of a grin
On his face. If he worried he hid it.
He started to sing as he tackled the thing
That couldn't be done, as he did it.
Somebody scoffed: "Oh, you'll never do that;

At least no one we know has done it";
But he took off his coat and he took off his hat,
And the first thing we knew he'd begun it.
With a lift of his chin and a bit of a grin,
Without any doubting or quiddit,
He started to sing as he tackled the thing
That couldn't be done, and he did it.
There are thousands to tell you it cannot be done,
There are thousands to prophesy failure;
There are thousands to point out to you, one by one,
The dangers that wait to assail you.
But just buckle right in with a bit of a grin,
Just take off your coat and go to it;
Just start to sing as you tackle the thing
That cannot be done, and you'll do it

A Smile-Author Unknown

A smile costs nothing, but gives much-

It takes but a moment, but the memory of it usually lasts forever.

None are so rich that can get along without it-

And none are so poor but that can be made rich by it.
It enriches those who receive, without making poor those who give-

It creates sunshine in the home,
Fosters good will in business,
And is the best antidote for trouble-

And yet it cannot be begged, borrowed, or stolen, for it is of no value

Unless it is given away.

Some people are too busy to give you a smile-
Give them one of yours-

For the good Lord knows that no one needs a smile so badly

As he or she who has no more smiles left to give.

If You Think You are Beaten-Walter D. Wintle

If you think you are beaten, you are.
If you think you dare not, you don't.
If you'd like to win but think you can't,
It's almost certain you won't.
Life's battles don't always go
To the stronger or faster man,
But sooner or later, the man who wins
Is the man who thinks he can.

Men Whom Men Condemn as Ill-Joaquin Miller

In men whom men condemn as ill
I find so much of goodness still,
In men whom men pronounce divine
I find so much of sin and blot,
I do not dare to draw a line
Between the two, where God has not.

Just One-Unknown

One song can spark a moment,
One flower can wake the dream
One tree can start a forest,
One bird can herald spring.
One smile begins a friendship,
One handclasp lifts a soul.
One star can guide a ship at sea,
One word can frame the goal
One vote can change a nation,
One sunbeam lights a room
One candle wipes out darkness,
One laugh will conquer gloom.
One step must start each journey.
One word must start each prayer.
One hope will raise our spirits,
One touch can show you care.
One voice can speak with wisdom,
One heart can know what's true,
One life can make a difference,
You see, it's up to you!

If I Had my Child To Raise Over Again-by Diane Loomans

If I had my child to raise all over again,
I'd build self-esteem first, and the house later.
I'd finger paint more, and point the finger less.
I would do less correcting and more connecting.
I'd take my eyes off my watch, and watch with my eyes.
I would care to know less and know to care more.
I'd take more hikes and fly more kites.
I'd stop playing serious, and seriously play.
I would run through more fields and gaze at more stars,

I'd do more hugging and less tugging.
I'd see the oak tree in the acorn more often,
I would be firm less often, and affirm much more.
I'd model less about the love of power,
And more about the power of love

Don't Quit-Unknown

When things go wrong as they sometimes will;
When the road you're trudging seems all uphill;
When the funds are low, and the debts are high;
And you want to smile, but you have to sigh;
When care is pressing you down a bit
Rest if you must, but don't you quit.
Success is failure turned inside out;
The silver tint of the clouds of doubt;
And you can never tell how close you are;
It may be near when it seems afar.
So, stick to the fight when you're hardest hit
It's when things go wrong that you mustn't quit.

Promise Yourself-The Optimist Creed

Promise yourself to be so strong that nothing can disturb
your peace of mind.

To talk health, happiness, and prosperity to every person
you meet.

To make all your friends feel like there is something in
them.

To look at the sunny side of everything and make your
optimism come true.

To think only of the best, to work only for the best, and expect only the best.

To be just as enthusiastic about the success of others as you are about your own.

To forget the mistakes of the past and press on the greater achievements of the future.

To wear a cheerful countenance at all times and give every living person you meet a smile.

To give so much time to the improvement of yourself that you have no time to criticize others.

To be too large for worry, too noble for anger, and too strong for fear, and too happy to permit the presence of trouble.

Follow Your Dream-by Amanda Bradley

Follow your dream.
Take one step at a time and don't settle for less,
Just continue to climb.

Follow your dream.
If you stumble, don't stop and lose sight of your goal
Press to the top.
For only on top can we see the whole view,
Can we see what we've done and what we can do;
Can we then have the vision to seek something new,

Press on.
Follow your dream.

My Comfort Zone-Unknown

I used to have a comfort zone where I knew I wouldn't fail.

The same four walls and busywork were really more like jail.

I longed so much to do the things I'd never done before,
But stayed inside my comfort zone and paced the same old floor.

I said it didn't matter that I wasn't doing much.

I said I didn't care for things like commission checks and such.

I claimed to be so busy with the things inside the zone,
But deep inside I longed for something special of my own.

I couldn't let my life go by just watching others win.

I held my breath; I stepped outside and let the change begin.

I took a step and with new strength I'd never felt before,
I kissed my comfort zone goodbye and closed and locked the door.

If you're in a comfort zone, afraid to venture out,
Remember that all winners were at one time filled with doubt.

A step or two and words of praise can make your dreams come true.

Reach for your future with a smile; success is there for you!

Start Where You Stand-Berton Braley

Start where you stand and never mind the past,
The past won't help you in beginning new,
If you have left it all behind at last
Why, that's enough, you're done with it, you're through;
This is another chapter in the book,
This is another race that you have planned,
Don't give the vanished days a backward look,
Start where you stand.
The world won't care about your old defeats
If you can start anew and win success;
The future is your time, and time is fleet
And there is much of work and strain and stress;
Forget the buried woes and dead despairs,
Here is a brand-new trial right at hand,
The future is for him who does and dares,
Start where you stand.

Playing The Game-Unknown

Life is a game with a glorious prize,
If we can only play it right.
It is give and take, build and break,
And often it ends in a fight;
But he surely wins who honestly tries
(Regardless of wealth or fame),
He can never despair who plays it fair
How are you playing the game?
Do you wilt and whine, if you fail to win
In the manner you think your due?
Do you sneer at the man in case that he can
And does, do better than you?

Do you take your rebuffs with a knowing grin?
Do you laugh tho' you pull up lame?
Does your faith hold true when the whole world's blue?
How are you playing the game?
Get into the thick of it - wade in, boys!
Whatever your cherished goal;
Brace up your will till your pulses thrill,
And you dare - to your very soul!
Do something more than make a noise;
Let your purpose leap into flame
As you plunge with a cry, "I shall do or die,"
Then you will be playing the game.

All for the Best-By Edgar A. Guest

Things mostly happen for the best.
However hard it seems to-day,
When some fond plan has gone astray
Or, what you've wished for most is lost
An' you sit countin' up the cost
With eyes half-blind by tears o'grief
While doubt is chokin' out belief,
You'll find when all is understood
That what seemed bad was really good.
Life can't be counted in a day.
The present rain that will not stop
Next autumn means a bumper crop.
We wonder why some things must be-
Care's purpose we can seldom see-
An' yet long afterwards we turn
To view the past, an' then we learn
That what once filled our minds with doubt
Was good for us as it worked out.
I've never know an hour of care
But that I've later come to see
That it has brought some joy to me.

Even the sorrows I have borne,
Leavin' me lonely an' forlorn
An' hurt an' bruised an' sick at heart,
An' though I could not understand
Why I should bow to Death's command,
That it was really better so.
Things mostly happen for the best.
So narrow is our vision here
That we are blinded by a tear
An' stunned by every hurt an' blow
Which comes to-day to strike us low.
An' yet some day we turn an' find
That what seemed cruel once was kind.
Most things, I hold, are wisely planned
If we could only understand.

Why Not You? By Steve Maraboli

Today, many will awaken with a fresh sense of inspiration.

Why not you?

Today, many will open their eyes to the beauty that surrounds them.

Why not you?

Today, many will choose to leave the ghost of yesterday behind and seize the immeasurable power of today.

Why not you?

Today, many will break through the barriers of the past by looking at the blessings of the present.

Why not you?

Today, for many the burden of self doubt and insecurity will be lifted by the security and confidence of empowerment.

Why not you?

Today, many will rise above their believed limitations and make contact with their powerful innate strength.

Why not you?

Today, many will choose to live in such a manner that they will be a positive role model for their children.

Why not you?

Today, many will choose to free themselves from the personal imprisonment of their bad habits.

Why not you?

Today, many will choose to live free of conditions and rules governing their own happiness.

Why not you?

Today, many will find abundance in simplicity.

Why not you?

Today, many will be confronted by difficult moral choices and they will choose to do what is right instead of what is beneficial.

Why not you?

Today, many will decide to no longer sit back with a victim mentality, but to take charge of their lives and make positive changes.

Why not you?

Today, many will take the action necessary to make a difference.

Why not you?

Today, many will make the commitment to be a better mother, father, son, daughter, student, teacher, worker, boss, brother, sister, & so much more.

Why not you?

Today is a new day!
Many will seize this day.
Many will live it to the fullest.

Why not you?

It's The Journey That's Important-By John McLeod

Life, sometimes so wearying
Is worth its weight in gold
The experience of traveling
Lends a wisdom that is old
Beyond our 'living memory'
A softly spoken prayer:
"It's the journey that's important,
Not the getting there!"
Ins and outs and ups and downs
Life's road meanders aimlessly?
Or so it seems, but somehow
Leads us where we need to be,
And being simply human
We oft question and compare...
"Is the journey so important
Or the getting there?"
And thus it's always been
That question pondered down the ages
By simple men with simple ways
To wise and ancient sages...
How sweet then, quietly knowing
Reaching destination fair:
"It's the journey that's important, Not the getting there!"

You Travel Through Life-Unknown

As you travel through life there are always those times

When decisions just have to be made,
When the choices are hard, and solutions seem scarce,
And the rain seems to soak your parade.
There are some situations where all you can do
Is simply let go and move on,
Gather your courage and choose a direction
That carries you toward a new dawn.
So pack up your troubles and take a step forward
The process of change can be tough,
But think about all the excitement ahead
There might be adventures you never imagined
Just waiting around the next bend,
And wishes and dreams just about to come true
In ways you can't yet comprehend!
Perhaps you'll find friendships that spring from new things
As you challenge your status quo,
And learn there are so many options in life,
Perhaps you'll go places you never expected
And see things that you've never seen,
Or travel to fabulous, faraway worlds
And wonderful spots in between!
Perhaps you'll find warmth and affection and caring
And somebody special who's there
To help you stay cantered and listen with interest
To stories and feelings you share.
Perhaps you'll find comfort in knowing your friends
Are supportive of all that you do,
And believe that whatever decisions you make,
They'll be the right choices for you.
So keep putting one foot in front of the other,
And taking your life day by day...
There's a brighter tomorrow that's just down the road -
Don't look back! You're not going that way!

Keep Them Close-Unknown

One day a mother died.

And on that clear, cold morning,
in the warmth of her bedroom,
the daughter was struck with
the pain of learning that sometimes there isn't any more.

No more hugs, no more lucky moments to celebrate
together, no more phone calls just to chat, no more "just
one minute."

Sometimes, what we care about the most goes away,
never to return before we can say good-bye, say "I Love
You."

So while we have it … it's best we love it .
And care for it and fix it when it's broken
and take good care of it when it's sick.
This is true for marriage … and friendships!

And children with bad report cards;
and dogs with bad hips;
and aging parents and grandparents.

We keep them because they are worth it,
because we cherish them!

Some things we keep -
like a best friend who moved away
or a classmate we grew up with.

There are just some things that
make us happy, no matter what.

Life is important, and so are the people we know.

And so, keep them close!

Count That Day Lost-By George Eliot

If you sit down at set of sun
And count the acts that you have done,
And, counting, find
One self-denying deed, one word
That eased the heart of him who heard,
One glance most kind
That fell like sunshine where it went-
Then you may count that day well spent.
But if, through all the livelong day,
You've cheered no heart, by yea or nay-
If, through it all
You've nothing done that you can trace
That brought the sunshine to one face-
No act most small
That helped some soul and nothing cost-
Then count that day as worse than lost.

Life-by Nan Terrell Reed

They told me that Life could be just what I made it
Life could be fashioned and worn like a gown;
I, the designer, mine the decision
Whether to wear it with bonnet or crown.

And so I selected the prettiest pattern
Life should be made of the rosiest hue
Something unique, and a bit out of fashion,
One that perhaps would be chosen by few.

But other folks came and they leaned o'er my shoulder;

Someone questioned the ultimate cost;
Somebody tangled the thread I was using;
One day I found that my scissors were lost.
And somebody claimed the material faded;
Somebody said I'd be tired ere 'twas worn;
Somebody's fingers, too pointed and spiteful,
Snatched at the cloth, and I saw it was torn.

The World Is Against Me-By Edgar A. Guest

"The world is against me," he said with a sigh.
"Somebody stops every scheme that I try.
The world has me down and it's keeping me there;
I don't get a chance. Oh, the world is unfair!
When a fellow is poor then he can't get a show;
The world is determined to keep him down low."
"What of Abe Lincoln?" I asked. "Would you say
That he was much richer than you are to-day?
He hadn't your chance of making his mark,
And his outlook was often exceedingly dark;
Yet he clung to his purpose with courage most grim
And he got to the top. Was the world against him?"
"What of Ben Franklin? I've oft heard it said
That many a time he went hungry to bed.
He started with nothing but courage to climb,
But patiently struggled and waited his time.
He dangled awhile from real poverty's limb,
Yet he got to the top. Was the world against him?
"I could name you a dozen, yes, hundreds, I guess,
Of poor boys who've patiently climbed to success;
All boys who were down and who struggled alone,
Who'd have thought themselves rich if your fortune they'd known;
Yet they rose in the world you're so quick to condemn,
And I'm asking you now, was the world against them?"

My Creed-By Edgar A. Guest

To live as gently as I can;
To be, no matter where, a man;
To take what comes of good or ill
And cling to faith and honor still;
To do my best, and let that stand
The record of my brain and hand;
And then, should failure come to me,
Still work and hope for victory.
To have no secret place wherein
I stoop unseen to shame or sin;
To be the same when I'm alone
As when my every deed is known
To live undaunted, unafraid
Of any step that I have made;
To be without pretense or sham
Exactly what men think I am.
To leave some simple mark behind
To keep my having lived in mind,
If enmity to aught I show,
To be an honest, generous foe,
To play my little part, nor whine
That greater honors are not mine.
This, I believe, is all I need
For my philosophy and creed.

Things Work Out-By Edgar A. Guest

Because it rains when we wish it wouldn't,
Because men do what they often shouldn't,
Because crops fail, and plans go wrong
Some of us grumble all day long.
But somehow, in spite of the care and doubt,
It seems at last that things work out.
Because we lose where we hoped to gain,

Because we suffer a little pain,
Because we must work when we'd like to play
Some of us whimper along life's way.
But somehow, as day always follows the night,
Most of our troubles work out all right.
Because we cannot forever smile,
Because we must trudge in the dust awhile,
Because we think that the way is long
Some of us whimper that life's all wrong.
But somehow we live and our sky grows bright,
And everything seems to work out all right.
So bend to your trouble and meet your care,
For the clouds must break, and the sky grow fair.
Let the rain come down, as it must and will,
But keep on working and hoping still.
For in spite of the grumblers who stand about,
Somehow, it seems, all things work out.

Influence-By Joseph Norris

Drop a pebble in the water,
And its ripples reach out far;
And the sunbeams dancing on them
May reflect them to a star.
Give a smile to someone passing,
Thereby making his morning glad;
It may greet you in the evening
When your own heart may be sad.
Do a deed of simple kindness;
Though its end you may not see,
It may reach, like widening ripples,
Down a long eternity.

Before You-By William Arthur Ward

Before you speak, listen.
Before you write, think.
Before you spend, earn.
Before you invest, investigate.
Before you criticize, wait.
Before you pray, forgive.
Before you quit, try.
Before you retire, save.
Before you die, give.

Do More-By William Arthur Ward

Do more than belong: participate.
Do more than care: help.
Do more than believe: practice.
Do more than be fair: be kind.
Do more than forgive: forget.
Do more than dream: work.

We Must-By William Arthur Ward

We must be silent before we can listen.
We must listen before we can learn.
We must learn before we can prepare.
We must prepare before we can serve.
We must serve before we can lead.

Be The Best of Whatever You Are-By Douglas Malloch

If you can't be a pine on the top of the hill,
Be a scrub in the valley-but be
The best little scrub by the side of the rill;
Be a bush if you can't be a tree.
If you can't be a bush be a bit of the grass,

And some highway happier make;
If you can't be a Muskie then just be a bass
But the liveliest bass in the lake!
We can't all be captains, we've got to be crew,
There's something for all of us here,
There's big work to do, and there's lesser to do,
And the task you must do is the near.
If you can't be a highway then just be a trail,
If you can't be the sun be a star;
It isn't by size that you win or you fail
Be the best of whatever you are!

May You Have-Unknown

May you have......
Enough happiness to keep you sweet,
Enough trials to keep you strong,
Enough sorrow to keep you human,
Enough hope to keep you happy;
Enough failure to keep you humble,
Enough success to keep you eager,
Enough friends to give you comfort,
Enough wealth to meet your needs;
Enough enthusiasm to look forward,
Enough faith to banish depression,
Enough determination to make each day better than
yesterday.

Profit From Failure-Unknown

The test of a man is the fight he makes,
The grit that he daily shows;
The way he stands on his feet and takes
Fate's numerous bumps and blows.
A coward can smile when there's naught to fear,
When nothing his progress bars;

But it takes a man to stand up and cheer
While some other fellow stars.
It isn't the victory, after all,
But the fight that a brother makes;
The man who, driven against the wall,
Still stands up erect and takes
The blows of fate with his head held high;
Bleeding, and bruised, and pale,
Is the man who'll win in the by and by,
For he isn't afraid to fail.
It's the bumps you get, and the jolts you get,
And the shocks that your courage stands,
The hours of sorrow and vain regret,
The prize that escapes your hands,
That test your mettle and prove your worth;
It isn't the blows you deal,
But the blows you take on the good old earth,
That show if your stuff is real.

Handwriting On The Wall-Unknown

A weary mother returned from the store,
Lugging groceries through the kitchen door.
Awaiting her arrival was her 8 year old son,
Anxious to relate what his younger brother had done.
While I was out playing and Dad was on a call,
T.J. took his crayons and wrote on the wall
It's on the new paper you just hung in the den.
I told him you'd be mad at having to do it again.
She let out a moan and furrowed her brow,
Where is your little brother right now?
She emptied her arms and with a purposeful stride,
She marched to his closet where he had gone to hide.
She called his full name as she entered his room.
He trembled with fear--he knew that meant doom
For the next ten minutes, she ranted and raved

About the expensive wallpaper and how she had saved.
Lamenting all the work it would take to repair,
She condemned his actions and total lack of care.
The more she scolded, the madder she got,
Then stomped from his room, totally distraught.
She headed for the den to confirm her fears.
When she saw the wall, her eyes flooded with tears.
The message she read pierced her soul with a dart.
It said, I love Mommy, surrounded by a heart.
Well, the wallpaper remained, just as she found it,
With an empty picture frame hung to surround it.
A reminder to her, and indeed to all,
Take time to read the handwriting on the wall.

Success-Unknown

Success is speaking words of praise,
In cheering other people's ways.
In doing just the best you can,
With every task and every plan.
It's silence when your speech would hurt,
Politeness when your neighbor's curt.
It's deafness when the scandal flows,
And sympathy with others' woes.
It's loyalty when duty calls,
It's courage when disaster falls.
It's patience when the hours are long,
It's found in laughter and in song.
It's in the silent time of prayer,
In happiness and in despair.
In all of life and nothing less,
We find the thing we call success.

The Most Beautiful Flower-Unknown

The park bench was deserted as I sat down to read
Beneath the long, straggly branches of an old willow tree.
Disillusioned by life with good reason to frown,
For the world was intent on dragging me down.
And if that weren't enough to ruin my day,
A young boy out of breath approached me, all tired from play.

He stood right before me with his head tilted down
And said with great excitement, "Look what I found!"
In his hand was a flower, and what a pitiful sight,
With its petals all worn - not enough rain, or too little light.
Wanting him to take his dead flower and go off to play,
I faked a small smile and then shifted away.
But instead of retreating he sat next to my side
And placed the flower to his nose and declared with
overacted surprise,

"It sure smells pretty and it's beautiful, too.
That's why I picked it; here, it's for you."
The weed before me was dying or dead.
Not vibrant of colors: orange, yellow or red.
But I knew I must take it, or he might never leave.
So I reached for the flower, and replied, "Just what I need."
But instead of him placing the flower in my hand,
He held it mid-air without reason or plan.
It was then that I noticed for the very first time
That weed-toting boy could not see: he was blind.
I heard my voice quiver; tears shone in the sun
As I thanked him for picking the very best one.
"You're welcome," he smiled, and then ran off to play.
Unaware of the impact he'd had on my day.
I sat there and wondered how he managed to see
A self-pitying woman beneath an old willow tree.

How did he know of my self-indulged plight?
Perhaps from his heart, he'd been blessed with true sight.
Through the eyes of a blind child, at last I could see.
The problem was not with the world; the problem was me.
And for all of those times I myself had been blind,
I vowed to see the beauty in life,
And appreciate every second that's mine.
And then I held that wilted flower up to my nose
And breathed in the fragrance of a beautiful rose
And smiled as I watched that young boy,
Another weed in his hand,
About to change the life of an unsuspecting old man.

Climb 'Til Your Dream Comes True-Helen Steiner Rice

Often your tasks will be many,
And more than you think you can do.
Often the road will be rugged
And the hills insurmountable, too.
But always remember,
The hills ahead
Are never as steep as they seem,
And with Faith in your heart
Start upward
And climb 'til you reach your dream.
For nothing in life that is worthy
Is ever too hard to achieve
If you have the courage to try it,
And you have the faith to believe.
For faith is a force that is greater
Than knowledge or power or skill,
And many defeats turn to triumph
If you trust in God's wisdom and will.
For faith is a mover of mountains,
There's nothing that God cannot do,
So, start out today with faith in your heart,

And climb 'til your dream comes true!

The Guy in the Glass-by Dale Wimbrow

When you get what you want in your struggle for self
And the world makes you king for a day
Just go to the mirror and look at yourself
And see what that man has to say.
For it isn't your Father or Mother or wife
Whose judgment upon you must pass.
The fellow whose verdict counts most in your life
Is the one staring back from the glass.
Some people may call you a straight shooting chum
And call you a wonderful guy,
but the man in the glass says you're only a bum
If you can't look him straight in the eye.
He's the fellow to please, never mind all the rest
For he's with you clear to the end,
And you have passed your most dangerous test
If the man in the glass is your friend.
You may face the whole world down the pathway of life
And get pats on the back when you pass,
But your final reward will be heartache and strife
If you've cheated the man in the glass.

The Challenge-by Jim Rohn

Let others lead small lives,
But not you.

Let others argue over small things,
But not you.

Let others cry over small hurts,
But not you.

Let others leave their future
In someone else's hands,

But not you.

My Wage-by Jessie B. Rittenhouse

I bargained with life for a penny,
And life would pay no more,
However I begged at evening
When I counted my scanty store;
For life is a just employer,
He gives you what you ask,
But once you have set the wages,
Why, you must bear the task.
I worked for a menial's hire,
Only to learn dismayed,
That any wage I had asked of life,
Life would have paid.

Watch-By Frank Outlaw

Watch your thoughts, for they become words.
Watch your words, for they become actions.
Watch your actions, for they become habits.
Watch your habits, for they become character.
Watch your character, for it becomes your destiny.

Equipment-By Edgar A. Guest

Figure it out for yourself, my lad,
You've all that the greatest of men have had,
Two arms, two hands, two legs, two eyes
And a brain to use if you would be wise.
With this equipment they all began,

So start for the top and say, "I can."
Look them over, the wise and great
They take their food from a common plate,
And similar knives and forks they use,
With similar laces they tie their shoes.
The world considers them brave and smart,
But you've all they had when they made their start.
You can triumph and come to skill,
You can be great if you only will.
You're well equipped for what fight you choose,
You have legs and arms and a brain to use,
And the man who has risen great deeds to do
Began his life with no more than you.
You are the handicap you must face,
You are the one who must choose your place,
You must say where you want to go,
How much you will study the truth to know.
God has equipped you for life, but He
Let's you decide what you want to be.
Courage must come from the soul within,
The man must furnish the will to win.
So figure it out for yourself, my lad.
You were born with all that the great have had,
With your equipment they all began,
Get hold of yourself and say: "I can."

Don't Dwell-Author Unknown

Don't dwell on what might have been or the chances you have missed.

Or the lonely nights that lie between the last time lovers kissed.

Don't grasp too hard the memory of the things that never came.

The door that did not open or the wind that killed the flame.
There is still time enough to live...And time enough to try
again.

Be Happy.

Our Deepest Fear-By Marianne Williamson

Our deepest fear is not that we are inadequate.
Our deepest fear is that we are powerful beyond measure.
It is our light, not our darkness that most frightens us.
We ask ourselves
Who am I to be brilliant, gorgeous, talented, fabulous?
Actually, who are you not to be?
You are a child of God.
Your playing small
Does not serve the world.
There's nothing enlightened about shrinking
So that other people won't feel insecure around you.
We are all meant to shine,
As children do.
We were born to make manifest
The glory of God that is within us.
It's not just in some of us;
It's in everyone.
And as we let our own light shine,
We unconsciously give other people permission to do the
same.
As we're liberated from our own fear,
Our presence automatically liberates others.

The Invitation-By Oriah Mountain Dreamer

It doesn't interest me what you do for a living.
I want to know what you ache for,
And if you dare to dream of meeting

Your heart's longing.
It doesn't interest me how old you are.
I want to know if you will risk looking like a fool
For love, for your dream,
For the adventure of being alive.
It doesn't interest me what planets are squaring your
moon.
I want to know if you have touched the center of your own
sorrow,
If you have been opened by life's betrayals,
Or have become shriveled and closed from fear of further
pain.
I want to know if you can sit with pain,
Mine or your own,
Without moving
To hide it or fade it or fix it.
I want to know if you can be with joy,
Mine or your own,
If you can dance with wildness
and let the ecstasy fill you to the tips of your fingers and
toes
Without cautioning us to be careful, be realistic,
or to remember the limitations of being human.
It doesn't interest me if the story you are telling me is true.
I want to know if you can disappoint another to be true to
yourself,
If you can bear the accusation of betrayal and not betray
your own soul.
I want to know if you can be faithless and therefore be
trustworthy.
I want to know if you can see beauty
Even when it is not pretty every day,
And if you can source your life
From its presence.
I want to know if you can live with failure,
Yours and mine,

And still stand on the edge of a lake and shout to the silver
of the full moon,
"Yes!"
It doesn't interest me to know where you live or how much
money you have.
I want to know if you can get up after the night of grief and
despair,
Weary and bruised to the bone,
And do what needs to be done for the children.
It doesn't interest me who you are, how you came to be
here.
I want to know if you will stand
In the center of the fire with me
And not shrink back.
It doesn't interest me where or what or with whom you
have studied.
I want to know what sustains you
From the inside
When all else falls away.
I want to know if you can be alone
With yourself,
And if you truly like the company you keep
In the empty moments.

Hidden Mystery-By Fred Burks

In the deepest depths of you and me
In the deepest depths of we
Lies the most beautiful jewel
Shining forth eternally
Within that precious jewel
Within that priceless piece of we
Lies a time beyond all time
Lies a place beyond all space
Within that sacred source of radiance
Lies a love beyond all love

Waiting
Waiting
Waiting
Ever so patiently
Waiting for you, waiting for me
Waiting patiently for all to see
The beauty that is you inside of me
The beauty that is me inside of thee
In the deepest depths of you and me
In the deepest depths of we
Lies the love and wisdom
Of all Eternity

Look Well to This Day-Anonymous, 50 B.C.

Look well to this day,
For it and it alone is life.
In its brief course
Lie all the essence of your existence:
The Glory of Growth
The Satisfaction of Achievement
The Splendor of Beauty
For yesterday is but a dream,
And tomorrow is but a vision.
But today well lived makes every yesterday a dream of
happiness,
And every tomorrow a vision of hope.
The Serenity Prayer
By Reinhold Neibuhr
God grant that I might have
The courage to change the things I can,
The serenity to accept the things I cannot,
And the wisdom to know the difference

Compassion-By WingMakers

Angels must be confused by war.
Both sides praying for protection,
yet someone always gets hurt.
Someone dies.
Someone cries so deep
they lose their watery state.
Angels must be confused by war.
Who can they help?
Who can they clarify?
Whose mercy do they cast to the merciless?
No modest scream can be heard.
No stainless pain can be felt.
All is clear to angels
except in war.
When I awoke to this truth,
it was from a dream I had last night.
I saw two angels conversing in a field
of children's spirits rising like silver smoke.
The angels were fighting among themselves
about which side was right,
and which was wrong.
Who started the conflict?
Suddenly, the angels stilled themselves
like a stalled pendulum,
and they shed their compassion
to the rising smoke
of souls who bore the watermark of war.
They turned to me with those eyes
from God's library,
and all the pieces fallen
were raised in unison,
intertwined like the breath
of flames in a holy furnace.
Nothing in war comes to destruction,

but the illusion of separateness.
I heard this spoken so clearly I could only
write it down like a forged signature.
I remember the compassion,
mountainous, proportioned for the universe.
I think a tiny fleck still sticks to me,
like gossamer threads
from a spider's web.
And now, when I think of war,
I flick these threads to all the universe,
hoping they stick on others as they did me.
Knitting angels and animals
to the filamental grace of compassion.
The reticulum of our skyward home.

That I A Better Person May Be-Author Unknown

Light that lies deep inside of me
Come forth in all thy majesty
Show me thy gaze
Teach me thy ways
That I a better person may be
Darkness that lies deep inside of me
Come forth in all thy mystery
Show me thy gaze
Teach me thy ways
That I a better person may be
Love that lies deep inside of me
Come forth in all thy unity
Let me be thy gaze
Let me teach thy ways
That I a better person may be

It Takes Courage-by Author Unknown

It takes strength to be firm,

It takes courage to be gentle.
It takes strength to conquer,
It takes courage to surrender.
It takes strength to be certain,
It takes courage to have doubt.
It takes strength to fit in,
It takes courage to stand out.
It takes strength to feel a friend's pain,
It takes courage to feel your own pain.
It takes strength to endure abuse,
It takes courage to stop it.
It takes strength to stand alone,
It takes courage to lean on another.
It takes strength to love,
It takes courage to be loved.
It takes strength to survive,
It takes courage to live.

May You Have Enough-by Fion Lim

May you have a healthy body,
To move around freely and roam wherever you desire to
go.
May you have good vision,
To enjoy all the beauty the universe has to offer you.
May you have good listening ears,
To hear all the mighty tales and incredible stories that
make up life.
May you have a good sense of smell,
To inhale in all the rich aromas and fragrances floating in
the air.
May you have a warm sense of touch,
To give out loving hugs and comforting pats.
May you speak with kindness from your heart,
To soothe someone's hurt and to uplift someone's mood.
May you have lots of laughter,

To brighten up someone's day and make a difference.
May you have lots of courage,
To go after your dreams and turn them into reality.
May you have lots of love,
To spread around and leaving this world a better place.
May you have enough to feel blessed,
And to share your gift of blessings with others too.

Self-Control-by Author Unknown

I've heard it said don't go to bed
while hanging on to sorrow,
you may not have the chance to laugh
with those you love tomorrow.
You may not mean the words you speak
when anger takes its toll,
you may regret your actions
once you've lost your self-control.
When you've lost your temper
and you've said some hurtful things,
think about the heartache
that your actions sometimes bring.
You'll never get those moments back,
such precious time to waste,
and all because of things you said
in anger and in haste.
So if you really love someone
and your pride has settled in,
you may not ever have the chance
to say to them again....
"I love you and I miss you,
and although we don't agree,
I'll try to see your point of view,
please do the same for me."

Seeking for Happiness-Ella Wheeler Wilcox

Seeking for happiness we must go slowly;
The road leads not down avenues of haste;
But often gently winds through by ways lowly,
Whose hidden pleasures are serene and chaste
Seeking for happiness we must take heed
Of simple joys that are not found in speed.
Eager for noon-time's large effulgent splendor,
Too oft we miss the beauty of the dawn,
Which tiptoes by us, evanescent, tender,
Its pure delights unrecognized till gone.
Seeking for happiness we needs must care
For all the little things that make life fair.
Dreaming of future pleasures and achievements
We must not let to-day starve at our door;
Nor wait till after losses and bereavements
Before we count the riches in our store.
Seeking for happiness we must prize this -
Not what will be, or was, but that which is.
In simple pathways hand in hand with duty
(With faith and love, too, ever at her side),
May happiness be met in all her beauty
The while we search for her both far and wide.
Seeking for happiness we find the way
Doing the things we ought to do each day.

The Things That Count-Ella Wheeler Wilcox

Now, dear, it isn't the bold things,
Great deeds of valor and might,
That count the most in the summing up of life at the end of
the day.
But it is the doing of old things,
Small acts that are just and right;

And doing them over and over again, no matter what
others say;
In smiling at fate, when you want to cry, and in keeping at
work when you want to play -
Dear, those are the things that count.
And, dear, it isn't the new ways
Where the wonder-seekers crowd
That lead us into the land of content, or help us to find our
own.
But it is keeping to true ways,
Though the music is not so loud,
And there may be many a shadowed spot where we
journey along alone;
In flinging a prayer at the face of fear, and in changing into
a song a groan -
Dear, these are the things that count.
My dear, it isn't the loud part
Of creeds that are pleasing to God,
Not the chant of a prayer, or the hum of a hymn, or a
jubilant shout or song.
But it is the beautiful proud part
Of walking with feet faith-shod;
And in loving, loving, loving through all, no matter how
things go wrong;
In trusting ever, though dark the day, and in keeping your
hope when the way seems long -
Dear, these are the things that count.

The Superwoman-Ella Wheeler Wilcox

What will the superwoman be, of whom we sing -
She who is coming over the dim border
Of Far To-morrow, after earth's disorder
Is tidied up by Time? What will she bring
To make life better on tempestuous earth?
How will her worth

Be greater than her forbears? What new power
Within her being will burst into flower?
She will bring beauty, not the transient dower
Of adolescence which departs with youth -
But beauty based on knowledge of the truth
Of its eternal message and the source
Of all its potent force.
Her outer being by the inner thought
Shall into lasting loveliness be wrought.
She will bring virtue; but it will not be
The pale, white blossom of cold chastity
Which hides a barren heart. She will be human -
Not saint or angel, but the superwoman -
Mother and mate and friend of superman.
She will bring strength to aid the larger Plan,
Wisdom and strength and sweetness all combined,
Drawn from the Cosmic Mind -
Wisdom to act, strength to attain,
And sweetness that finds growth in joy or pain.
She will bring that large virtue, self-control,
And cherish it as her supremest treasure.
Not at the call of sense or for man's pleasure
Will she invite from space an embryo soul,
To live on earth again in mortal fashion,
Unless love stirs her with divinest passion.
To motherhood she will bring common sense -
That most uncommon virtue. She will give
Love that is more than she-wolf violence
(Which slaughters others that its own may live).
Love that will help each little tendril mind
To grow and climb;
Love that will know the lordliest use of Time
In training human egos to be kind.
She will be formed to guide, but not to lead -
Leaders are ever lonely - and her sphere
Will be that of the comrade and the mate,

Loved, loving, and with insight fine and clear,
Which casts its searchlight on the course of fate,
And to the leaders says, 'Proceed' or 'Wait.'
And best of all, she will bring holy faith
To penetrate the shadowy world of death,
And show the road beyond it, bright and broad,
That leads straight up to God.

You Are My Butterfly-by Tanja Cilia

You Are……… My Butterfly
You brought color to my life….
You helped me to select the sweet from the bitter
And savor the moment.
You showed me how to take things lightly
You helped me soar above
My worries.
You helped me spread my wings
And notice the flowers.
You are my butterfly, and I love you.
You showed me it's true that if
You chase a butterfly, away he flies;
But if you sit still, he brushes your cheek
With his wings and changes the
Monochrome vistas of grey
Into a suffusion of color.
Never were poppies so crimson
Or daffodils so yellow
As now.
Green apples and honey
Mint and liquorice and ginger, and
Stamens of the honeysuckle
Were never so real.
You are my butterfly.
Diving into the cool water
Feeling the warmth of a puppy

Touching an empty cocoon
Listening to the rain
Seeing the sun set
Hearing the rustle of leaves
Were never so aesthetic and sensual
As they has become since I
Met you.
For you are
My Butterfly.
You are my inspiration, the love of
My Life.
My Butterfly.

Courage-by Fion Lim

Courage is not only gifted to the few brave ones,
It is something that lies within you,
Where you can draw upon its strength and power,
In times of crisis, fears and decisions.
Courage is not something mysterious or unattainable,
It is something that you can exercise in your daily life
choices,
You can let it bring to you untraveled paths,
And make you more conscious and aware of your life.
Courage does not have to roar to be heard,
It does not mean being totally fearless and being
invincible,
It could mean taking actions, taking risks, taking a stand,
Standing up for yourself, standing by your choices,
And sticking to your dreams when others jeered.
Courage could be the will to live in spite of the struggles,
In spite of your fears and phobias, in spite of what others
said,
In spite of criticisms and disapproval, in spite of mistakes
and failures,

In spite of everything that stands between you and your
dreams.
Courage could mean trying over and over again when you
failed,
Admitting that you are sorry when you are in the wrong,
Saying I love you when your love is angry,
Having a baby when the idea of being a parent scared you,
Listening to your heart when others called you a fool,
Following your dreams even when others discouraged you,
And staying true to yourself when others want you in
another way.
Hold steadfast to your dreams, your heart and yourself,
And courage will not abandon you,
But follows you whenever you choose to go.

Hope You Enjoyed The Poems!

Visualizing Your Future

(Video Transcription)

It's time to talk about the subconscious Death Wish. I know quite a few of you in this room have met Leonard Orr because Lynn had him out to speak at her PI group.

How many know who Leonard Orr is or has met him? Okay about half-okay- so this is a subject that he became best known for and he started these rebirthing seminars about removing the Death Urge.

What is the Death Urge? We've talked about it a little bit- the idea that we become programmed by our civilization and our subconscious that we're expected to die-at a certain time.

You're told that you're supposed to retire when you get to your 50s you're supposed to be planning your retirement- not saying don't plan to save money I mean that's a good thing to do-but we're told that you're supposed to retire, live for a decade or two, then go to retirement home and then kaput.

That's been programmed into us-and it doesn't have to be.

So this is the common understanding we're taught from birth we're fated to mature, have a few years of healthy life, and die of old age.

I put together a list of different specifics that were taught okay-so we're supposed to physically slow down starting in our 30s, become less mobile in our 60s, and pretty much bedridden in our 80s, If you're not doing that you're not going with the flow here-all right you're going to disappoint a lot of the health insurance companies. You're not using their services enough.

That as we get old we're not supposed to still be attractive or healthy-that's only for younger people.

Advertising to start planning for your own funeral-God I hate that-How many times I heard on the local radio station that -come on up to Forest Lawn you've only got a few years left-is what they're implying- so get one of our nice funeral packages so we can put you to put you to bed there in another few years.

I mean how incredible is it that you know you're supposed to be programmed to die-that really gets to me.

Retirement planning-Yes I try and plan for retirement financially not because I want to die but because I want to quit working right-except doing stuff like this-- and so you only look at a time frame into your 80s because you're not going to need any more money after that anyway. Social Security and Medicare again implying you're not going to be able to take care of yourself--you're going to be too old and frail and a lot of people let themselves become that way.

You're going to lose your memory and your ability to think clearly- again not that what we believe but here are the assumptions of the world surrounding us.

Old people are ugly. You've not got anything interesting to do after your kids move away and you retire from your job therefore quit.

And obviously if you have an attitude that the life's not worth living that's going to affect you. How many times have you seen an older married couple where one spouse dies and the other spouse sickens and dies within six months or a year. I remember a really dramatic example when I was a paper boy as a teenager and there was this nice old couple in their 80s. They were both with white hair and they were always very very friendly to me and very outgoing and the husband got sick and died and the wife who was so outgoing and a little overweight-within six months she turned into frail skin and bones and just passed away. She had lost her will to live. So that's a very common thing. I mean it's pretty accepted that's a very common thing.

And medical care being rationed from old people. I don't want to get into my politics but that's another thing-okay I'd like to see what examples you think you can come up with of how we're programmed to die.

Can you guys think of anything? Taking drugs-okay programming today right there-they need to take a lot more medicine and everything of course those into making more -yeah more times exactly-that's another life is in preparation of death is that when you're this age you're going to not be able to see very welcome you and late and that they just reject all of these different things that are going to happen so and then people buy into it.

I'm 54 in this body and every year for the last 10 years people have been saying to me "how come you don't have glasses yet" you know you need glasses. I don't need glasses. I mean my sight isn't what it used to be but I don't need glasses. Any other ones? I know a couple times on the radio I heard them say you have cancer? Talk about programming a death wish.

How many times have you talked to somebody who says "I don't want to live to 100-there's not that much I'd want to do at that age" I mean they've already decided this is the span of life I'm going to live and there's not much more I really want to do so therefore forget it.

Because they have internalized and they expect that by the time they get to any age of 70 or 80 they're not going to held to have the health or the ability to do anything. So naturally they assume there's no point going on.

We have to change that. We have to learn to internalize the things we're doing this weekend so that we realize that we can be healthy. We can enjoy things. We can have multiple careers. I mean when I think about going out to three hundred, five hundred, a thousand years, I think about the list of things I'd like to do which includes having multiple professions. Doctor, I don't know about lawyer, don't mean to offend any lawyers in the room—I would like to have multiple professions.

I'd like to go everywhere in the world, and I'd like to start taking some trips out into space, and in the solar system. I'm sure there's a lot more interesting things to see out there too.

I would like to be married several more times if my partner doesn't last-not that I wanted to have a serial marriages or all that but you understand where I'm going.

There's just so much life to live, if you enjoy it. I mean I'd like to be creative. I would like to do lots of things. I'm trying to make this into a new career for myself. Why not?

When I think about teaching longevity and physical immortality, really the older you get the more credibility you have. So by the time I get to be a hundred I'm going to be able to fill up stadiums. Okay? If I'm 150 or 200 years old you know they'll just listen to my every word, because this is one profession where the older you get the more credible you are. Right?

So anyway, these are some of the things to think about when we're talking about the Death Wish. So you can remove the Death Wish; this contributes to your physical renewal.

Dennis and Lynne and I have talked a lot about this. That the approach to do this is not to negate negative imagery. Because that only focuses on the negative imagery. It is to focus on positive imagery. Positive visualization in believing you can stay healthy and live forever. And don't pay attention to what people tell you in actuarial statistics. Probably the biggest reason I think that we accept we have to have a short lifespan is because insurance companies and other companies that publish actuarial statistics. And they say you're just not going to live any longer than this. The odds of living longer than 80 or 90 years is very small and only a small proportion of the population is going to do that. So don't even bother.

It's all pre-programmed there's nothing you can do about it okay- so we have these expectations set in us-so think about it-just from a pure psychological basis-forget all the spiritual stuff-forget all that healthy energy stuff that we've talked about this weekend.

But if you are programming yourself so that you can only live a limited span-that's the way you're going to live your life- that's the way you're going to expect your health to be that's where you're going to plan everything with that goal in mind. That by 70 or 80 that's it.

So just by changing your attitude you can extend your life. Really. Forget all the rest of it-just by changing your attitude.

Okay now I know you all know what visualization is so I'm not going to spend time focusing on this. I wasn't sure how many in the audience would be familiar. You are all pretty familiar with the techniques. The main thing I'd like to focus on before we get into the next exercise is that that you need to remind yourself that the key to successful visualization is not that you will do something, but that you are doing something-that you're in the now.

Okay and that's what we're going to focus on in the next exercise that you're in the now when we do this. So this is going to be an exercise and visualizing your mortal future.

So you should start preparing yourself and relaxing. Close your eyes if you would. Start relaxing using breathing or whatever you feel most comfortable with. I'll give you a couple minutes for that.

In this exercise we're going to visualize our ages going forward at different future ages. I want you to start thinking about happy scenes that you want to visualize yourself being in. That may occur at different ages of seeing your friends, or activities, or a location you would want to come back to.

Now I want you to visualize that you're a hundred years old. You are in the scene. The people in the scenery are around you. You can feel what temperature it is. You can see the light in the sky or the ceiling of the room or building that you're in. You also smell the scene and you see everything vividly. You are there. You can look around and see details such as trees, or buildings, or paintings, and what your friends or family you're doing. Your body feels healthy. You can tell that you're youthful. Your solid belief in your own physical immortality has been paying off for a while now. You enjoy different sports or activities that you find fun. Being with friends and family. You may have a profession or an artistic endeavor which you enjoy doing and you like to keep doing.

Now we're going to shift forward. You're now 200 years old. It's the 23rd century. Maybe your lifestyle changed.

Maybe you went to a simpler life and location. Or maybe you decided you wanted to live in the city. But again you're going to see your surroundings very vividly and the scene that you enjoy.

Feel all five senses. Your sight, your hearing, your smell, your touch. What do you see? What do you hear? What do you smell and taste? What do you feel? Who is with you? How much of things changed. You're actually there. You're in the 23rd century. It's probably a mixture of the old and the new. We're probably exploring the solar system. Science is taking great leaps forward and people are realizing their spirituality more often every day.

You're now 500 years old. It's the 25th century. You may have traveled into the solar system or to a planet around another star. Life goes on and you're in a community. Maybe other immortals like you who have similar interests. You may have taken on a new profession or are in an artistic mode you've never tried before. By now you may have learned a secret of different abilities like how to teleport yourself and let you live totally in the now.

Let's look around and see what's there. You feel very strong and healthy as you usually do and you've been healthy and physically stable for centuries. You don't think too much about the past. You think about how much you enjoy the now and how much you enjoy the things you're going to do. Because as far as you're concerned living every day is a joy. There's no need to change that.

You might want to project yourself further. To a further distant age that's somewhat incomprehensible to us. But you've been evolving through time and now you're enjoying that age, and the friends, and family you've made have taken this journey with you.

To new locations or to a state we can't even imagine. But yet existence goes on because the consciousness of life in the universe is eternal. Visualize for a couple of minutes and then you can come out.

Okay thank you. Come out of it. I hope you enjoyed that one. It's a kind of a little different tack-kind of going through the time stream we're doing a lot of visualization but we want to try and take it in different tracks and work on different issues.

Positive Affirmations

(Video Transcript)

Okay-the last major thing we have on today is to talk about Harry Gazes books. As I mentioned in the beginning today, I've done a lot of research on different people throughout the ages have talked about physical immortality.

We've talked about longevity and we're going to cover a lot more material tomorrow; but I found this is an interesting book by a gentleman named Harry Gaze written in 1904. And he was a philosopher and teacher in practical metaphysics, and he published numerous books on metaphysics. He believed in a lot of different principles about the body and the conscious cooperation with the life force of the body is something that will help vitalize you. Help keep you excited. Help keep you young. And that again getting to part of our subject we're going to cover tomorrow in terms of the Death Urge. It's related to that-that you can prevent the conditions which cause physical death-they can be prevented by having the right subconscious image and the right thoughts about your body.

And he had a variety of exercises for that. So first we'll look at the golden rules he had, and then we're going to go through some affirmations together verbally about this. He had a lot of different things we talked about which are similar to this, but realize that as a son of God, you're an heir to God's immortality here and now. You can claim your birthright.

The only reason-and I'll get I have some examples tomorrow-but one of the biggest reasons we think we have to die is because we're told that. We're told that by commercials. We're told that by the way people talk about their lives. And I've got some specific examples for tomorrow about that.

I don't want to steal my thunder from that. But realize that your body is the expression of your mind and you can you can attune it to the infinite spirit. And when you do that your body's health naturally becomes smoother, becomes clearer, and becomes more peaceful.

Again getting back to LI-Ching-Yung we talked about having a peaceful heart. Okay-just some of the same principles.

Nature constantly renews your body. I think the period is every few months or six months, almost all your cells are recycled. So by being able to have the right attitudes, have the right energy, eat the right foods, you can renew your body. There's no reason it has to stay unhealthy.

Here's another point that I thought was really good that so I put it in red-Eternal Youth uses a harmony and positive cooperation of continuous growth and the law of attraction. So in other words what are we attracting to us? Are attracting to us health and vitality? Or are we attracting to us a feeling that the end is coming.

It's really a lot about our attitude. Okay so these are affirmations of positive outlooks. And what I want to do and get to the first page here--these are almost A through Z. I don't know if there's 26 of them there's quite a few-but what I want to do is I'm going to read them and as I read them I'd like you guys to repeat them because the idea is to internalize these affirmations of a positive attitude.

Not to talk about a negative or negative of a negative but internalize a positive and get rid of the negative. Let's start okay…..

Adaptation-Whenever essential I adapt myself readily to more perfect change.

Adjustment-I give myself freely to wise spiritual mental and physical adjustment.

Beauty-I realized that the beauty of enduring youth is as deep as an innermost recesses of the soul.

Buoyancy-in every thought nerve and muscle I expressed the perfect buoyancy of joyous youth there's no reason that I have to feel tired. I can feel full of joy and full of youth.

Confidence-I cheerfully react to all conditions with the boundless confidence of youth. The youth are confident people that are in their 20s or teens they know they can lick the world. We sell off and lose that when we get older. So let's get that confidence back.

Courage-increasingly attain the natural courage of the strong and vital you. When you're healthy, when you feel positive, you have courage to do things.

Creativeness-Creativeness is a quality that we can have at any age but it's also something that sometimes we lose when we think negatively or lose our positive outlook on life. So the Divine Spirit everywhere and in and through me inspires me with keen creativeness.

Flexibility-and elasticity the word used. Again a lot of people that are old tend to think in channels. They tend to think certain things are impossible. We need to break that, we need to break those boundaries. My sense of freedom and flexibility of mine and its correspondence in daily elasticity.

Energy-Obviously it's important. We have to have the energy and vitality in our life. So that we want to do things. So that we want to enjoy our life. There's so much to enjoy in the world. So let's be positive about that. My whole being is vitally energized with the radiant life of the Divine Spirit.

Flexibility-Similar to elasticity. I joyously affirm the quality of flexibility in every cell muscle or an artery of my being. There's no reason that if we're getting older we can't be as flexible both physically and mentally as those who are younger than us.

Freshness-Bathing in the Commonality of pure spirit, I am fresh as the dawn of the day. There's no reason that you can't feel as fresh as a newborn. Okay, It doesn't matter your age-it's all a matter of attitude.

Gracefulness-By wise exercise, relaxation, visualization, and nourishment, I maintain the gracefulness of youth. We don't have to be old and ugly. We can be vital, we can be alive, we can be young, and we can have the gracefulness of a child.

Happiness-I can't overemphasize the importance of happiness, and happiness comes from within. Happiness is something that the Spirit gives us in abundance. All we have to do is see that it's there. We're going to talk about happiness a lot more tomorrow, but happiness as related to love and enlightenment. But it's a critical factor, so let's cover that. I realize that the true spring of happiness is within me.

Initiative-The spirit of initiative and wise adventure really motivates and activates me. Initiative is something that we can do at any point in our life. We don't have to decide just because we're older that we can't do new things, that we can't learn new things, that we can't have new creativity. We can take all the initiative we want for the things that are important in our lives.

Joy-The joy of eternal youth is my daily light and inspiration. This can be something that's joyous for everyone. Why would you want to live a long time if you can't have joy in your life? You have to have joy in your life to make it worthwhile. That's part of what we're talking about here. That's part of what this whole weekend is about. It's about experiencing joy in your life because you don't find any very old very unhappy people. They are happy, and they enjoy their lives; otherwise they wouldn't want to go on with it. So the joy of eternal life or eternal youth is my daily light and inspiration.

Related to that is loveliness, not just in a physical sense-but that you love yourself. The loveliness of ever renewing youth is the expression of love, loving, and lovable qualities.

Newness-Every day and every moment my body is being made new in every cell, molecule, and Atom. We can live in the present. We can imagine we are not only imagined but be realizing that we are renewing from moment to moment. Okay

Optimism-We have to have optimism in our lives. Optimism is what gives us the ability to get out of bed in the morning, and to enjoy life rather than letting ourselves be dragged through the day. Okay Optimism is all about having confidence in yourself to do new things. To enjoy life. To create things. To be positive with people. To build relationships. So Optimism-I look joyously forward with the spirit of youthful optimism.

Progressiveness-I'm not talking politics. I'm a progressive, conscious, purposeful, and individual factor in my evolution. In other words, I'm going to let myself evolve the way I want to. My life is going to evolve the way I directed. I'm going to be progressive in deciding what I want to do and what my future is going to be rather than letting circumstances control me.

Purity-I see life with the eyes of childlike purity blended with power. Purity is again something that comes from having the spirit in your life. The more that you have that the purer you will feel. The more your motivations will be positive. The more you will have love in your life. Purity is something we have as a child but we tend to lose it as we grow older because of the pressures of daily existence. But that's not to say we can't reclaim it.

Radiance-I'm radiant with a light, life, and love of infinite wisdom. Yes, you can be radiant. You can have the radiance of God's light in your life. I don't mean to sound like a preacher. But we're talking about how you want to be. How you want to let the infinite spirit penetrate you and be within you and radiate to other people. You want to be a light in their lives. You don't want to be just sucking energy. You want to be somebody who stands out. Who has the energy and the vitality to radiate all around to other people, and heat them up spiritually. So radiance.

Receptivity-Knowing that I'm a child of God. I am at all times receptive to the highest inspiration. So part of this is being receptive to new concepts. Being receptive to new ideas which most people poopoo;

which they say are ridiculous; or you're insane to think that. So being receptive, opening your mind to new concepts, and new ways of thinking is also important.

Rejuvenation-That's what we're here for. I'm devoted and consecrated to all habit habits that rejuvenate and heal.

Renewal-I'm ever renewing, an ever unfolding expression of infinite life. We are constantly renewing. We need to realize that. We need to live that. Renewal

Responsiveness-As the years unfold I maintain my full free responsiveness to the best in life. I will participate. I will be involved. Go ahead responsiveness.

Unfoldment-I'm open, receptive, and responsive to new growth and unfoldments. We are unfolding as spiritual beings in this life. We're continuously growing if we're not growing we're stagnated. Everybody needs to grow. Even when they think they're totally enlightened, there's probably still room to grow. So by being open to unfolding, we are going to have a healthier, longer, happier life. Unfoldment

Versatility-I joyously express the creative spirit in me and the versatility that tempers youth with experience. Let's do that one.

Vitality-I think, speak, free exercise, relax, and nourish my mind and body for increasing vitality. We want to be vital. We want to be alive. We want to have more energy with people looking at us and acting asking themselves-- how do I get to be like that person? How do I have the energy that person has?

Youth-I realize that the fountain of eternal youth like the kingdom of God is here and now within me. And not just in terms of our immortal soul but in terms of the thousands of youth and the bodies we have today.

Finally-Zest-My thoughts, speech, and action are all radiantly animated with the youthful zest in living. I want to have a zest for life. I don't want to just go through life and exist. I want to really enjoy it. I want to have all the qualities that we talked about here. I want to be able to just enjoy my life. I want to be able to enjoy relationships with other people and have love in my life. I want to have a great time. Zest

Okay-Well thank you for going through all that-that was a little bit of work but i hope you liked it.

Additional Affirmations

(Transcribed from Audio file)

All the things I require-come to me.

I constantly receive more than what I require.

I have a bank account with more than enough.

I am an abundant individual.

I produce abundance in all that I say and do.

I accept abundance.

I receive and am open to receive all abundance that comes.

I draw abundance to myself today and each day. I'm successful.

Everything I do turns into success.

I'm filled with success.

My success is contagious. Others like it, seek it, and respect it. I draw in confident minded people to me.

I draw all things favorable to myself.

I'm really fortunate to work at what I love to do.

I make powerful and enjoyable business relationships.

And many of my business contacts are now my friends.

I'm a confident and positive individual, and confident and positive persons gravitate towards me daily.

I recognize what I obviously am, and what I like in personal relationships.

I'm attracting powerfully positive and healthy individuals into my life.

I'm caring, smart, supportive, loyal, and fun to be with.

I feel completely at ease and comfortable with all types of individuals.

I'm winning in all of my relationships.

I'm a positive and valuable contributor to all of my relationships.

I possess complete power to articulate my thoughts and feelings to everybody, and I express myself wisely.

I'm sure of my ability to do what is necessary to better my life.

If I make errors, I'm able to give myself the benefit of the doubt.

I feel worthy as an individual.

I'm able to take risks and try new things without concern. I feel great about the way I do my job.

I have compassion for myself and the way my life has developed.

I'm deserving of all of the good things in my life. I'm glowing with health and wholeness.

I behave in ways that promotes my health more each day. I deserve to be in perfect health.

I'm highly motivated to exercise my body, because I find exercise as fun.

I love nutritious healthy food, and I love eating fresh foods and veggies.

I'm healthy since my practices are healthy.

I release the past so I can create health now.

I produce health by producing love, understanding, and compassion.

Summary

As you can see, the Life Urge can be modified from death oriented to life oriented.

We don't have to be programmed to expect to die at a certain age. Our subconscious mind can help our longevity by being focused on positive life experiences and continuing vitality.

We can also re-energize ourselves with new inspirations.

We can control our positive and negative beliefs in our subconscious and need to realize that we have this ability to expect to live longer and happier lives.

www.ingramcontent.com/pod-product-compliance
Lightning Source LLC
Chambersburg PA
CBHW031226250726
48655CB00005B/1826